"Do you not know that your body is the temple (the very sanctuary) of the Holy Spirit Who lives within you, Whom you have received (as a gift) from God? You are not your own, You have been bought with a price (purchased with a preciousness and paid for, made His own), So then, honor God and bring glory to Him in your body" (1 Cor. 6:19-20 AMP).

I was inspired to write Temple Care as I observed people in the church gaining weight over the years. Christianity is the number one faith in America. Those stats say to me, the body of Christ is overweight to morbidly obese.

As I researched what the Word (Bible) said about the Creator's diet law/plan for His created, I realized many are lacking knowledge about it, or are in disobedience to "doing it", causing various health and social problems. God first designed a garden equipped with our food and herb source for health. Thereafter, created and placed humanity in it's midst. God later gave precise instruction's to the "REDEEMED" for personal and public health.

During the above process, I discovered that the State of Indiana, where I reside, at the time of the research in 2004, according to The Center of Disease Control (CDE), was the third most obese State in the United States. That said to me that as ministers of the gospel, we must not only be balanced in our teaching of the entire Word, we must also lead in every way by our example.

We are not just spirit, we possess a soul and we live in a body. God desires for His present earthly Temple (our body) to be healthy, so our spirit can navigate it to complete the will of God.

TEMPLE CARE

The enemy used humanity's food source, fruit, to
accomplish their first fall. It worked then, so
he's trying it again! Has food become a
weapon of mass destruction? If
all else fails, follow God's
diet law/plan!

REV. DR. STEPHANIE JORDAN

Temple Care
ISBN 978-098256340-3
Copyright © 2009 by Stephanie Jordan

Library of Congress Control Number: 2009938652

Published by
Knowledge Network Publishing
A Division of Knowledge Network
1211 Manhattan Street
Michigan City, Indiana 46360
www.knownetmc.com

CONTENTS

ACKNOWLEDGMENTS

It takes a team effort to fully actualize a research project; their act of assisting, encouraging and loving is immeasurable. To the following people and more, I am indebted. I acknowledge Heather Couch who patiently and professionally typed the manuscript while excitedly awaiting the next chapter. The love and support from Dr. Michael Messina, Rev. Gerald Glover, Dr. RoyEtta Quateka-Means, Dr. William Dixon, Dr. Kim Yancey-James, Dr. Percy Johnson, Dr. Maurice Ndukwu, Kathy Krachinski, Dr. Mary Taylor, Roxy Karnes, Diane Carter, Dr. Morven Nyaiyaye, Dr. Vidya Kora, Jerry Jones and Amy Rosa. My mentor Rev. Dr. Peggy Way and Faculty Advisor, Rev. Dr. Emma Justes for their direction and correction. For the formal assistance of Brenda Harvey, Dr. Carey Ransone, Dr. Lisa Hendricks, Dr. Danny Sardon and Dr. Karen Edwards, toward the success of the Temple Care, Back to Basics Workshop. To Margaret Mizia, who continued typing the manuscript without missing a beat with that same care and professionalism during the interim when Heather's grandma was ill. The prayers and support of Pastor Hoffman, First Lady, Sister Lorraine Hoffman and my entire River of Life Church family in Michigan City, IN, which has kept me going much like the Energizer Bunny. St. Anthony Memorial Medical Center in Michigan City, IN, for

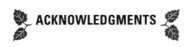 **ACKNOWLEDGMENTS**

the formal contributions and resources for the Workshop and toward my entire seminary journey. To Mandi Eggert who typed promotional letters. For John Kessler and Mark Lesniewski, my managers, who allowed me time off to write, and to my co-workers who filled in during my absence. To Father Larry Henry, who gave me articles on obesity. To Sister Mary Gerard, who constantly encouraged me. Sister Elizabeth Ann who assisted with the history of the hospital. To Countryside Christian Center for so lovingly allowing me to have access freely to the church library for resources. For the prayers of my ministerial associations—The Michigan City, Indiana Ministerial Alliance, Rhema Ministerial Association International, Full Gospel Chaplaincy and the Association of Professional Chaplains, I am in appreciation.

DEDICATION

To Jesus Christ, my Lord and Savior and inspirer of this work.

To my children, Misty M., Aina R., and Kushinda T., and grandchildren, this legacy demonstrating obedience to God.

To my grandmother, the late Rev. Etta Mae Morris, who exemplified Christ, and my mother, Genevieve Morris-Davis, who by her discipline enabled me to obey God.

INTRODUCTION

This story is about recovering the health of America. In planning and implementing this program, I demonstrated the possibility of positive work between church and hospital. Both are concerned about God's humanity; their quality of life issues are universal. The focus was on the pandemic of obesity, with a particular concern for the dietary history and dynamics of the African American community.

To accomplish this, I had to define the pandemic, demonstrate a constructive dialogue between scripture and contemporary medicine and look at the particular history and culture of food in the African American community. While this is a universal issue, I have a particular concern for the African American.

Therefore, this book shows church and hospital can successfully cooperate in dealing with this pandemic, and demonstrate a feasible dialogue between modern medicine and Scriptural perspective on human health. I am dealing with the controversial issue of Leviticus, Chapter 11, verses 1-12. These verses direct humanity toward beneficial sources of meat to eat.

Chapter 1 speaks to the issue of obesity in America. Churches and hospitals have consciously come together,

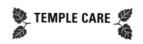

recognizing that humanity is spirit, soul and body and must be treated as such by each discipline. My spiritual autobiography will trace the seed that germinated for this project. The context became dual with both church and hospital ministries. However, it was at this point when the new passion was birthed. It became crystal clear through the synergy that it was a mandate from God for me to do my share to assist with changing the obesity stats in America for the better!

Chapter 2 demonstrates the ministry model for Temple Care. It describes the research it took to actualize the project. The aim was to scientifically demonstrate God's reasoning for dietary food laws/plans.

Chapter 3 covers the Biblical foundation for this work. It exegetes the Scriptures that form the foundation on which the research is built. It speaks to holistic care, spirit, soul and body. A breakdown of the Temple in the wilderness, to the heavenly temple and Jesus as temple, paves the way for one to understand how accepting Jesus as Lord enables one's body to become that temple where the Holy Spirit resides, to be revered and cared for as the Creator designed. It addresses clean and unclean meat. The chapter closes using the example of four particular Scriptures that have often been used to say the particular isolated Scripture is saying something it really is not.

Chapter 4 covers the Theological Foundation that speaks to information on the subject gained from some of our theological forefathers and foremothers, as well as other authors who have researched the Biblical diet and compared it to

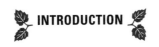

contemporary scientific data. The Bible and science are on one accord, with regard to dietary benefits and disasters.

Chapter 5 is the Historical Foundation, which was most exciting for me. It shares what was actually eaten during Biblical times, from what the Israelites ate in the wilderness, what Jesus ate and what was discovered from archaeological digs. It all points to the fuel that was designated for humanity in the handbook (Bible).

This section speaks to the African American slave diet and the history of "soul-food," as it relates to some of the diseases African Americans are afflicted with today. It also addresses hormones, antibiotics, preservatives, pesticides, and more that goes into processed meats etc., and calls for public action for it to be stopped.

Chapter 6 pertains to the Theoretical Section of Temple Care, which is motivation. Understanding the theory is a motivating factor. Motivation is especially beneficial from one who can relate. Knowledge is foundational; one can only work with that which is known.

Chapter 7 is a guide to duplicate the *Temple Care Back to Basics, 21-day Workshop*. It will suggest the assistance you will need for its success. Included is a printed version of my power point presentation that I used as an introduction to the workshop.

MINISTRY FOCUS

The ministry model is the relationship of Temple Care (See Bible), to improved health status for individuals afflicted with obesity. I will be using the Biblical metaphor for developing a wellness model with scientific understanding to encourage a lifestyle change for the human creature. In the Bible, the human is presented as whole: spirit, soul and body. Hospitals have come to realize this and now have Chaplains on the medical team to minister to one's spiritual needs. On the other hand, pastors have come to understand one's body has been neglected and therefore must also be addressed inclusively so they have congregational nurses teaching wellness programs.

I will be adding to this African American dietary concerns, as well as some of the new brain research that will contribute to a deeper understanding about food addicts. Addiction in the scientific community is not simply "sin." It contributes to the whole working of the human organism.

The foundational aspect of this project was birthed in 2004 after being pregnant spiritually for several years with

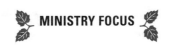

what I believe to be a mandate from God to minister to the overweight/obese congregants in the church and participants from a nearby hospital. During that incubation period, the concern for me was, "Would a message regarding obesity be received from one who is 'now' a size eight?"

The program will be implemented into the body of Christ (inviting obese clients from the nearby hospital) as part of the foundational teaching for new believers and the re-education of present members by the Word, with scientific backing for better understanding. It is anticipated this will begin a new cycle of holistic care. Body weight will decrease and a personal spiritual relationship with God will surely soar. The Christian church must lead by example.

I have concluded that, because Christianity is the larger percentage of American society, this renewal of mind and lifestyle change will have a profound impact on first the surrounding neighborhood and thereafter abroad. The hospital is the pulse of the community. The various diseases in the area are first counted in the hospital and reported to the health department to determine what diseases or situations are on the rise around us to be aware of. Those stats include obesity and diseases which are directly related to it.

I observed the congregation over the years increase in body fat. I kept praying for them, and the ministry call became clear. I am to be one of the instruments assigned to be part of the solution. I was reminded of a quote Dr. Lewis Baldwin cited from Dr. Martin Luther King Jr., regarding prayer. This is an illustration of the inclusiveness of prayer. Dr. King says, ". . . insisting that prayer must always be

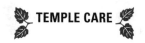

combined with hard work, intelligence, and sustained action."[1] With that said, a dream and a prayer without acting on it will never come to fruition.

When it's time for an infant to be birthed into the world, its mother has no say-so. I received the courage to deliver the message on Temple Care with the support of the senior pastor, and it was well received. The Word says, "My people (the Christians) are destroyed for lack of knowledge . . ." (Hosea 4:6). The Christian churches have a serious issue of obesity that must be addressed. According to recent stats from the American Obesity Association,

> The number of adults who are overweight/obese has continued to increase. Currently 64.5 percent of U.S. adults, age 20 and older, are overweight and 30.5 percent are obese.[2]

Most medical professionals define obesity in men as 25% or more body fat, and women with 30% or more are obese. It dawned on me that if Christianity is the largest faith in the U.S., "according to the Major Religions Ranked by size,"[3] does that mean that Christians are the most obese? Has food become a weapon of mass destruction, spiritually targeted at the Christians? Humanity's food source in the Garden of Eden (the interpreter's choice was a red apple) in the beginning was used to cause separation between God and humanity by their disobedience. Could it be this obesity epidemic is simply a continuation of that disregard of direction? Dr. Sharon Sneed, author of the *Love Hunger Action Plan* says,

> Today one out of every two Americans wants to lose weight. And at least 25 percent need to lose weight for

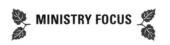

medical reasons. This constitutes an absolute epidemic of out-of-control fat cells.[4]

Biblical diet and rules have certainly been one of the most neglected areas by the body of Christ. Leviticus Chapter 11, verses 1-8, has been one of the most controversial. It's as though it is not a part of the canon. Of the top two faiths,

Christianity is ranked 33% and Islam is second at 21% and third is listed as non-religious, consisting of; agnostic, atheist, etc., and those answering to "none" hold the third place at 16%,[5]

This poses a concern. Of the Christians, one should exclude the 7th Day Adventists, where the larger percent adhere to a healthy diet, and so do the Muslims. "On the Major Religion pie scale, Judaism ranked 0.22% and no. 12 on the list."[6] Although low on the scale, most adhere to a strict diet.

There is a particular concern regarding the higher rate of African Americans having diseases, such as high blood pressure, diabetes, heart conditions and CVA (cerebral vascular accidents, strokes), to name the main effects from eating a high fat diet. This diet has been passed on generation after generation and adopted as culture, with most not understanding the true significance of its origin of survival. It appears to have become an addiction under the name of "soul food," a relationship that soothes some of the pain associated with societal stressors that the African American has endured over the generations.

I recall a sign of prosperity in the African American community at one time was when one could afford to buy

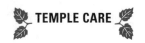

steak. An outward "sign" of one having moved up is a "prosperity belly" (a protruding abdomen). The gentleman would rear back, unbutton his coat and rub his expanded waist to display how well he has been eating.

Most who are addicted to food either do not realize it or have not accepted the fact that "food" is their addiction which, as with any other habit, has to be faced before one can be truly liberated. With substances such as drugs, alcohol, cigarettes, illicit sex and others, one can separate oneself through a program and work through the healing process. With food, one has to eat to live; food is ever before us. Eating less is a much longer withdrawal process.

I have been a registered nurse for 40 years and, therefore, had experience in almost every facet of nursing, including behavioral medicine, before accepting the call to ministry. It has been my experience, nicotine addicts were the most difficult to work with. The curiosity with food for me was, "Does the brain respond the same to food as it does to drugs?" because the behavior is so similar. Robert Mathias, a writer from the National Institute on Drug Abuse (NIDA), wrote an article titled, "Pathological Obesity and Drug Addiction Share Common Brain Characteristics." In the report, Mathias noted,

> Reduced brain activity of dopamine, a naturally occurring substance that modulates feelings and pleasure, may contribute to obesity as well as drug addiction, a NIDA-funded study suggests. The study found that the brains of obese individuals have relatively few of the nerve cell components called D2 receptors through which dopamine acts to stimulate

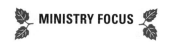

pleasurable feelings from basic activities such as eating and sex. Individuals with this deficiency may need to overeat to get a feeling of gratification from food, the researchers say. Because a deficit of the same receptors has been implicated in addiction to cocaine, heroin, and other drugs of abuse, the researchers suggest that it may be linked to a range of compulsive behaviors.[7]

The mind must be renewed. That knowledge could save one's mind from metaphorically being wasted or from literal atrophy. A Milwaukee study revealed that,

Obesity increased the risk of brain atrophy in women. Using brain scans after tracking weight gain in women over nearly a quarter century, researchers made a disturbing finding: as the body gets larger, the brain gets smaller.[8]

The above information confirms for me that food addicts also need help, and most cannot do it alone as they become discouraged and eat more, getting larger or are up and down in size, not consistent. In-patient programs for the obese should be as common today as the 30-day programs are for other addictions, if we are to really help.

I have a dream this 21-day program will turn into an in-patient program for the obese/morbidly obese. Dr. Fern Kazlow and most researchers agree "it takes 21 days to create/break a habit."[9] During that time, the residents will receive the knowledge and loving support they need from a staff that has "been there" (once obese) to help them jump-start a new lifestyle of activity and diet. The weight of the client will not be an issue as long as they are able to walk in. That is because

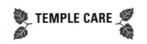

there will be physical activities, such as active games, walking, ballroom dancing and water aerobics, that will be segments of the program. In the situation of the Christian, one would be encouraged to develop a deeper relationship with Jesus, who is their higher power.

Stress is a main culprit of addiction. Therefore, it will be covered along with rest and diet. Pritchett Price calls stress, "The invisible epidemic. Antibiotics can't touch it. The microscope can't even spot it. It's rapidly spreading, and almost everybody's feeling the effect."[10]

Whatever one uses to ease the pain of stress could easily become a painkiller, if the stressor is not removed first. That anesthesia could be coffee, nicotine, sex, alcohol, drug of choice, i.e. prescription from the doctor or street drugs, food, work, sleep and more.

This project will now trace its origin in my spiritual autobiography. I will identify the depth of the problem, grounded in scriptural understandings, and develop and implement a program I am calling Temple Care.

Spiritual Autobiography

I am multicultural, raised African American. My father was the first African American pyro-meter man employed at A. Finkle and Sons Steel Mill, which is presently in operation on Chicago's north side. My mother was a homemaker and strict disciplinarian. I am the third born of six siblings, five of whom are living, and I am the first girl. My oldest brother died at six months to pneumonia. My mom wanted me and

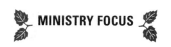

my siblings to attain the kind of education my parents did not have; therefore, we attended parochial schools. I was born, raised and remained in Chicago until I attended Bible School in Broken Arrow, OK, from 1990-1992. I came to Michigan City, IN on March 8, 1999, in preparation for marriage, so I thought. However, I gave birth to a dual ministry instead.

Seed of My Faith

The seed of my faith came from my maternal grandmother and mother. My grandmother was a solid Christian and a doer of God's Word. She was very humble with little to say. She never mentioned the sexism women, especially single, godly women, face in ministry. However, she resisted. I learned of her resistance to sexist treatment through stories from my mom.

As a student in the Catholic school system, we were compelled to attend Mass. After Mass on Sunday, we would attend my grandmother's church, "The Upper Room." She was founder and pastor. In retrospect, a female pastor in the 1950s was almost unheard of. Nevertheless, she lived a lifestyle that was exemplary of Christ, and her relationship with God kept the family centered.

I was fifteen when my grandmother looked at me with that "piercing through your spirit stare," and said in a soft, but matter-of-fact-tone, "Stephanie, God has a call on your life!" I could feel the presence of God and probably started running from the call as soon as she completed the sentence. I turned away moving my head from side to side as if to say,

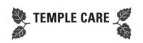

"No!" I said, "I want to be a nurse, God don't want everyone to preach!" To the day my grandmother died, she never mentioned it to me again. When she died, I was holding her hand and attempted CPR. I believe I received the baton at that time.

Werner Starks is quoted in James Cone's book, *God of the Oppressed,* which speaks about influences that are part of our development of thoughts, ideas and beliefs. Stark says, "We see the broad and deep acres of history through a mental grid . . . through a system of values which is established in our minds before we look out onto it, and it is this grid which decides what will fall into our field of perception."[11] I believe one of the functions of the "mental grid" is to develop a personal and unique way to customarily view and operate in the world. I clearly understand my thought mechanisms or "grids," including those that pertain to theology, are based on my grandmother's authority, my personal experience as an African American woman and the things I have discovered and learned while on my educational journey.

Birth of Ministry Passion

The seed of passion for *Temple Care* today was planted unknowingly when I was an overweight teen. I was much more developed than my peers with full breasts, hips and thighs. Some called me "pleasingly plump," which was another word for fat in 1958.

No one ever knew the physical or psychological pain I endured. I suffered silently, as most overweight and obese people do. I did not share my story until later in adult life to

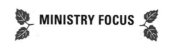

encourage a teen that was overweight. My family said in retrospect they never saw me as overweight; they thought I "looked good" however, no one ever asked how I felt.

The question was never asked why I walked strange at times. I had inner thigh abrasions that would not heal because of the constant friction of my thighs rubbing as I walked. The wounds were so raw (angry, it is called in the medical field) they were like a cancer sore. I had to wear a special undergarment to prevent the rubbing so I could walk naturally and not be wide-legged to prevent their touching and therefore pain. I was made aware by my physician the only way the abrasive thighs would heal completely was if I lost twenty-five or thirty pounds, and that I did.

My family thought I was dieting for modeling purposes. They observed and laughed as I bumped my hips and thighs on the floor to the tune of whatever exercise program was on TV. I continued to wear the special undergarment until I lost the weight. I accepted as a teen that maintaining a certain weight had to become a lifestyle, not a quick diet. I did not want to ever regain the weight and pain that accompanied it.

I did become a registered nurse. I married my childhood sweetheart and soon became concerned about getting pregnant. Some of the women in my family looked like sumo wrestlers after they had a baby. When I became pregnant with our first daughter, I began to weigh my meat portions. I also went on long walks daily, not only for the exercise, but to help with an easier delivery. I managed to gain fewer than 25 pounds with each of the pregnancies. I have maintained a size eight since 1967.

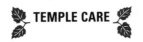

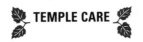

TEMPLE CARE

My concern was with my husband, who was addicted to "soul food." My distress was regarding the high fat content and high blood pressure, diabetes and other diseases that result from consuming high fat on a regular basis.

I stopped eating pork in 1972, "not" because I was taught the Levitical food laws because I had not heard of them, but because I wanted to grow old gracefully without high blood pressure or something else related to fat.

I was employed at that time with the Chicago Reclamation District as an industrial registered nurse. I had sent a few overweight African American men home with high blood pressure. I sent a young African American man in his early 30s to the hospital by ambulance with stroke-level blood pressure. He confessed he was on blood pressure pills. However, the pill rendered him impotent; therefore, he did not take the medication over the weekend so he could function sexually and forgot to resume taking them.

I called his wife to let her know I sent her husband to the hospital, and to encourage her to put him on a low-fat diet. She became emotional over the telephone, sharing that they had some of their most explosive arguments when she attempted to remove him from soul food, replacing it with low fat meals and salads. She said, "He is addicted to soul fool," and if she does not prepare it, he might lose control.

Having heard various stories like, "I'm not a rabbit, feed me," I must admit I did not know how to approach my husband, who was also addicted to "soul food." There is a time and place for everything, so I waited for the perfect time. That time was not at the dinner table; it was after

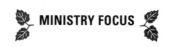
making love, while lying in his arms. I simply said, "Sweetheart, I would like for us to preserve this. I desire for you to continue to function like this for many years to come, and the only way that we can accomplish that is to change our diet to low fat, to avoid high BP and/or other related health problems."

We were in our late 20s. I shared some of the horror stories about men in their early 30s with high blood pressure because of a high fat diet. I mentioned the medication they took to lower their blood pressure unfortunately rendered them impotent. I truly had his undivided attention after that statement. I suggested we do it gradually, eliminating pork first. It went so smoothly; I could have given a class on "how to wean your husband from soul food."

He took the lead and we gradually became vegetarians. I presently eat salmon and white fish, and an abundance of fruits, vegetables and herb supplements. We juiced fresh vegetables daily. It was at that time when my health was at its best. I was myopic at that time; I consequently had to wear prescription lenses. After a year of drinking carrot juice daily, I went for my yearly eye exam and was told I had 20/20 vision. My response was, "Doc, didn't you see me walk in here with thick glasses on my face?" He said, "Well, what have you been doing since your last visit?" I thought for a minute, and it came to me that it was the carrot juice and dietary changes. That was in 1973. I started wearing .75 magnifying reading glasses (which is very mild, the lowest over the counter reading glasses start at 1.0) when I started Bible school in 1990 as a result of reading fine print. Today, I continue to wear reading glasses only. God's fruits,

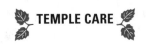

vegetables, and herbs are healing. I believe that is the reason He placed us in the garden surrounded by all we needed to sustain life abundantly.

My husband and I were raised in Chicago as Christian. Nonetheless, neither of us had developed a relationship with the Lord prior to our marriage. To be honest, I didn't realize it then, he was my god. Through his quest to get to know God, was drawn to Islam. My body and soul were pulling on me to acquiesce to the religion, to be with him; however, my spirit would not.

I therefore was forced to choose between my God, whom I did not really know personally and nevertheless had a reverential fear of, and my man whom I loved as much as life itself. I learned later that reverential fear I experienced was the beginning of wisdom. The pain of our divorce was the catalyst to a true relationship with my Lord and Savior, Jesus Christ.

Journey to Obedience

Along that journey, I attended Rhema Bible Training Center because I was insatiably thirsty for God and not getting enough knowledge of Him. Six months before graduation, I prayed and asked God what He would desire for me to do after graduation that would give Him the most glory. Through a dream, I received, "SEEK CHAPLAINCY!" I smiled and said, "Oh God, I never thought of that. You are keeping me in the hospital in another position."

During Christmas break, I sought a position as a hospital chaplain and was graciously informed I needed Clinical Pastoral Education (CPE). So, in the summer of 1992, my CPE journey began with a basic unit at Mercy Hospital in Chicago. My CPE residency was done at Christ Hospital and Medical Center in Oak Lawn, IL, from September 1993 to August 1994. One of the greatest assets I came away with is the ability to disagree agreeably with respect, perhaps for such a time as this. God prepares us along the way for the mission.

I was ordained at Rhema Bible Church in Broken Arrow, OK, by the Rev. Kenneth Hagin Sr. on March 23, 1994. I worked as a part-time, on-call chaplain for the Advocate System (Christ Hospital) from 1994-1999. I have been a full time chaplain at St. Anthony Memorial Medical Center in Michigan City, IN, since April 3, 2000.

I am in two separate ministries; however, they flow together in the same community. The hospital ministry is one of presence and compassion. I am also an assistant pastor to the Rev. Roderick Hoffman at River of Life Missionary Church in Michigan City, IN, near the hospital. The church and hospital are multicultural. The church is non-denominational; the hospital patients and employees are a mixture of all faith beliefs. I deliver the message at the church approximately once a month and sometimes when pastor is out of town. I also take the message of *Temple Care* to the community churches.

A seminary degree was necessary to become certified as a chaplain. However, I did not want to go back to school. I finally accepted the fact I was in disobedience to God by not

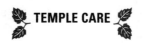

attending seminary because it was a requirement to complete the journey I perceived God called me to do. Without asking God what seminary, I quickly registered where a CPE student attended, Chicago Theological Seminary, fall 2000, graduated May 2005. I believe God reveals His divine plan for our lives one step at a time as we are obedient to and have completed the previous instruction.

Two of the most painful areas of growth for me in seminary were inclusive language (gender distinction) and attempting to fit myself into a particular methodology in ministry. I do not consider inclusive language inappropriate. I welcome it. For me, it is change and change is a process that takes time. I had been accustomed to "man" in the Word of God to mean both man and woman and had been comfortable with it. However, I welcome the distinction between male and female instead of assuming the male as the model for the species as tradition would have it.

My difficulty came primarily with the language for God. That is where my feelings of what some call heresy came in. I am comfortable calling God He or Father. However, if I'm around someone who is not, I found relief in words I feel comfortable with that would not lessen God's position as Godhead. In the place of the male pronoun (which is where the offense usually comes) for God the Father, I use Creator, for the Son, Redeemer, the Holy Spirit is neutral. I am at peace because the name defines who it represents. If language is a hindrance to one getting close to God, the language that is necessary should be used. I believe our language (God-talk) is as different as our fingerprints. However, just as God understands our various native

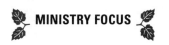

tongues, God unites with us where we are in our particular God-talk. After all, the relationship is personal.

The other area I struggled with was my ministry methodology. Before seminary, I was simply "a woman of God." However, in my final position paper, I had to label myself with a title that speaks to my style of ministry. I am an African American woman from a history of multi-cultural influences within my family that has affected what I believe and how I see and understand the world. This affects my thinking because clearly the different cultures of my mixed heritage have levels of privilege. Therefore, one who is mixed with African American is automatically placed on the lowest level. The sources of this quote came from personal experiences, such as not being served in a restaurant in the south and on the outskirts of Chicago, IL, in 1960 because I'm an African American. It has opened my eyes to the seriousness of humanity's unloving social constructs of racism and drew me closer to God's unconditional love. My background has also inspired me in what I have started to believe about God and what I believe about how God is present in the world. Therefore, the theological methodology that best expresses some of my theology is Womanist Theology, and it helps ground my passion for Temple Care.

I will speak briefly to Womanist Theology, because Alice Walker's definition is more fitting to my call to ministry. Part of her definition says, "A womanist is one who is serious, loving and committed to the survival and wholeness of entire people, male and female" (Musser & Price, 540.) Entire encompasses all of the human race. I minister to all cultures and faiths as a hospital chaplain and as an associate pastor.

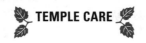

Much of Womanist Theology really is common sense and has roots in the things our mothers, grandmothers and great-grandmothers instilled in us based on their life experiences, passed on so that our people can continue to survive and encourage other men and women. My call is to pass the good news on to all of humanity that God leads me to.

Alice Walker approaches life in her Womanist Theology. She took the above common-sense approach to life and the world and connected it back to the things she had been taught through the women who walked before her. Some African American female Theologians piggybacked on those ideas and beliefs and used them to create a theology that also celebrates the uniqueness of African American women, especially with respect to relationships with God. My mother continues to share stories about how gracefully my grandmother lived through racism, sexism and classism as a pastor. From time to time as I go through the same and share with her, it may trigger her memory of something similar my grandmother also endured. A staunch Womanist would or may argue my language. However, we would be in one accord with relying on the Bible as the principle resource, using it as a tool to liberate by approaching the interpretation from a contemporary perspective.

Since graduation from CTS, I have completed the necessary requirements and, as of June 2006, I am a board certified chaplain with the Association of Professional Chaplains. As a hospital chaplain and an associate pastor, I have earned the respect of the various community clergy and residents across all faiths and I value that highly.

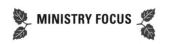

Culmination of the Journey

The passion seed for better temple care (body) has been planted, watered and developed at the United Theological Seminary by my professional associates, peer group and mentor. The aim was to develop a book and a workbook that will aid in the transforming of an obese unhealthy society to a slimmer, healthier one, while simultaneously earning a Doctorate Degree through research in the ministry. It is my hope that the residents of the State of Indiana will move from the number three position on the list of most obese states in the U.S. to a healthier position. It is my desire that the Temple Care Work Book will become a world changer, although I am well aware of my limitations and the complexities of change.

Context Analysis

My ministry context is dual. I have been a full time staff chaplain at St. Anthony Memorial Medical Center in Michigan City, IN, for the past nine years. I am also an assistant pastor to the Rev. Roderick Hoffman, at River of Life Church. Both ministries are located in the city approximately one mile or less in proximity of each other, therefore blending and flowing together in the same community.

Chaplain

There is no other hospital in Michigan City. There was one called Memorial; however, the Sisters purchased it and

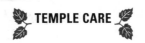

demolished the building. The present name then became St. Anthony Memorial. There are approximately 48,000 residents in Michigan City, IN. The hospital is also a trauma center. There is a heliport atop the new building above the emergency room, which has 20 rooms, a padded room and a decontamination room. There is a newly opened cardiac center with the latest state-of-the-art diagnostic noninvasive equipment. Open heart surgery is now being performed there. Our birthing suites look more like five-star hotel suites.

The hospital celebrated 100 years of service to the community in 2003. Sister M. Valeria and Sister M. Genevieve were selected by the Sisters of St. Francis at their mother house in Lafayette, IN, to come to Michigan City, IN, to organize and assume charge of St Anthony Hospital. They arrived on July 2, 1903 with $34.00, a mission, a focus and faith that God would provide.

The first benefactors were Lydia Bluett, who gave an entire block, and John H. Barker, owner of a freight car factory that employed 2,200 men, who donated $10,000 for the new facility. Although not a Catholic himself, he wanted the hospital to be conducted by the Catholic sisters. The mansion Mr. Barker's family lived in still stands. It has become a Michigan City historical site.

Unfortunately, one of the founding sisters, Sister Valeria, died in 1906 as a result of head injuries sustained in an elevator accident. The hospital has served the same area since 1903. They have continued building, rebuilding and remodeling since then. The first one had the capacity for 75 semi-private small rooms. It was 153 feet long and 45

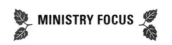

feet wide. It had a basement and three stories. Today, we have accommodations for 162 spacious private rooms with a sofa bed so loved ones can spend the night.

The Sisters believe in holistic care, spirit, mind (soul) and body. They further believe one's faith plays an important role in the healing process. I flow in and out ministering to people of various faiths, respecting them all by God's direction. Management of the hospital is oriented around God. The mission is to continue Christ's ministry from a Franciscan perspective, which is Respect for Life, Fidelity to our Mission, Compassionate Concern, Joyful Service and Christian Stewardship.

The staff and patient population are culturally diverse along with varied faiths. The immediate area surrounding the hospital is residential with the same cultural percentage as stated above. The community encompassing the residential area is the business and downtown district. That is where the banks, library, lawyers' offices, Wal-Mart, restaurants, shopping malls, etc., are located.

I also conducted a one-month sampling of the patient population's religion and the number of times the staff chaplain visited. Catholics were no. 1. None was no. 2, with Baptist being no.3.

None usually represented those who were bitter for some reason with organized religion or simply burned out for one reason or another. Listed under other included atheist, agnostic and denominations with fewer than five visits in the month, with most visits being only one or two times. Included in other were Muslim, COGIC, UCC, NAZ, AOG and

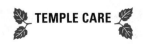

Apostolic of those who said they were Protestant or Christian believers in various degrees of relationship. The unknown status did not respond.

I am the first African American chaplain to have been hired in the 100-year history of the hospital's existence. When I was hired on April 3, 2000, there was a Methodist, 2 Lutherans, a priest and two Sisters, one of which was the manager to the department. I am presently the only full-time non-Catholic chaplain on staff. My relationship with God was solidified under the nondenominational church.

One of my ministry gifts is that of presence. It is a one-to-one crisis ministry, with the patient, their family, friends and staff. Presence not only entails simply being there, body and soul, it also includes being attentive to the situation without an agenda responsive to the direction of the Holy Spirit.

Birth of a New Passion

I believe the church and especially the hospital are the heartbeat of the Community and my ministry encompasses both. My graduate degree is nursing. Therefore, as I observed more and more around me, people in the church and elsewhere in the city who were obese/morbidly obese, a passion began to develop in me to help. At first, I simply began to pray for them. God was preparing me for such a time as this.

I don't like to simply preach/teach about a problem without a solution in mind for hope to solve it. I said to myself, where do I lovingly, tactfully begin? I began recruiting some of the other nurses in the church to do blood pressure screening. I thought that was a good place to start since many who have high blood pressure don't know it. It may be found when one is having a medical crisis, such as heart attack, stroke, a migraine headache, accumulated stressors or some other type of emergency.

There were a couple of members who knew they had high blood pressure for years, who were encouraged to seriously work on lowering it to avoid future kidney problems. There were a few with borderline high blood pressures. They were inspired to exercise, change their lifestyle eating habits and eat to live, not the reverse.

I did not want to wear two hats in the church, that of assistant pastor and nurse, simply because there are other nurses in the congregation. However, I had the passion to do something about the unhealthy physical state of some of the members.

I thought I would ignite someone's desire by talking about the congregational nurse program St. Anthony Memorial sponsors. I talked about how the congregational nurse kept a finger on the pulse of the congregation. In doing so, they knew what to do for upkeep and prevention.

Once the teaching needs have been assessed, then one in that field of expertise would be recruited to teach a class on the subject. An example would be, for diabetes teaching, someone from the Diabetes Association would be asked to speak. They usually have an assortment of many books on the subject that are very helpful. A dietitian can also help with balancing meals. I also mentioned how good our nurse

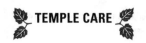

educator is at the hospital who may be willing to teach on needed subjects.

It was simply not the time to recruit a congregational nurse. However, I sensed the church in some way needed to address the sensitive issue of obesity. After all, we are not just spirit. We have a soul and a body to care for. They are connected and only separated at death. God addresses the whole person in the Word; therefore, we must also as ministers of the gospel of Jesus Christ. We must not only teach the Word, our lifestyles must exemplify it, especially leadership, spirit, soul and body.

It was clear to me God was unfolding this new mandate for me to do. God has a precise plan and a purpose for each of us individually that we must pursue, "for the gifts and the calling of God are irrevocable" (Rom. 11:29). God is such a gentleman; He takes us step by step as we obey. "…that you may prove what is that good and acceptable and perfect will of God" (Rom. 12:2). As God's plan is unfolding, it gets more and more exciting. It's usually something we didn't think we'd be doing, and especially being excited about it.

When that passion has been ignited and bursts into a flame, that is what drives one to complete it. When one has been given a controversial subject, such as I have, that passion is what keeps you going, knowing that the Word will back you. Again, Clinical Pastoral Education has prepared me to disagree respectfully for such a time as this. It took many, many years for America to get to this state of obesity; therefore, it will take some time to reverse.

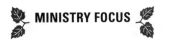

Assistant Pastor

I believe the passion seed to help the obese was being watered as I prayed for the obese around me. However, it was not totally revealed until later. I began to spend more time encouraging those who were obese or morbidly obese whenever I was impressed to do so by God. It became clearer through a sermon titled Temple Care that I was motivated to deliver at my home church, River of Life Missionary Church, Michigan City, IN. The church is also multicultural and youth culture conscious.

We are incorporated with the 501C3 tax-exempt status. The church is governed by a board of elders of which I am also a member. The Bible is the source of our activities and ministries.

"Three segment's of scripture are used to govern the Missionary Church; The Gospels, the Book of Acts, and the Epistles."[12]

I am an assistant pastor to Rev. Roderick Hoffman. He is married to Lorraine, who is the epitome of a pastor's wife.

They have two sons. The oldest, Roscoe, is praise leader and he is able to play many instruments except the horn. Joel, the youngest, plays saxophone. Lorraine sings, and pastor can play many instruments and sings as well.

Most men are not taught to be celibate until marriage. However, Roscoe and Joel were raised under that mandate. At the age of 29, on June 13, 2009 Roscoe, a chaste man, married Adele, also a virtuous woman. His brother Joel, was his BEST man.

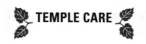

The church history began for the Hoffman family in August 1988 when they arrived at O'Hare Airport in Chicago from South Africa. Pastor said the only other person they knew there was God. He settled in Gary, IN, where he served a Southern Baptist Church. His salary was $350 a month plus a "monthly miracle."

The pastor appears to have a church-planting gift. River of Life Missionary Church is the second church he has pioneered since his arrival. Both churches are debt free. He is a 1992 Moody Bible Institute graduate.

In 2001, Rev. Hoffman was called to Michigan City, IN, where they started having services on their back porch. The pastor's focus is mainly street people who seemed to have lost their direction in life. He spends a lot of time identifying with those who are hurt and sharing that he was once an alcoholic, and how God brought him out, of addiction.

The mission statement is to reach the marginalized in our society with the life-transforming message of Jesus Christ, and to introduce them to a balanced life in the Spirit. His vision is to shatter every barrier and stereotype: to cross every cultural, financial, social and denominational line so ignorance will be obliterated by our central theme— Jesus Christ!

I was invited to the church by a member who was a patient in ICU, as I ministered to her. I visited the church and became a member months later. Thereafter, I became a board member and an assistant pastor.

The church is located within one mile from the hospital in a residential neighborhood. Encompassing the area is the same business district that surrounds the hospital. The area encircling the church is composed of 10% African American, 78% Caucasian (60% from Polish Catholic descent), 10% mixed culture families and 2% Hispanic. Of the above numbers, 65% are homeowners and 35% rent. The socioeconomic makeup of the above is 20% retired, 50% skilled and 30% professional. There are two neighborhood bars and one elementary school.

The cultural make-up of River of Life Church is 36% African American, 61% Caucasian and 3% Hispanic. The socioeconomic makeup is 40% professional/business owners, 40% skilled laborers, 12% retired, 6% unemployed/disabled and 2% are stay-at- home (domestic engineers) moms.

I selected a multicultural church because it was the type of setting where I began to develop a relationship with God. The Bible school and seminaries I attended had people from around the globe, and my heritage is multicultural.

The church neighbors have their thoughts about this new work that is developing in the neighborhood. The wife of one of the Caucasian residents was a patient in the hospital. As I was visiting her in the hospital, he mentioned the church. I did not know him; however, he knew who I was as a result of observing the activity around the church. They are in their 80s and have lived there since the birth of the church and have seen all of the prior pastors come and go over the past 50 + years, with Rev. Hoffman being the first African American pastor and the congregation being of mixed cultures.

He said with joy he has never seen so much love displayed, people of all colors, hugging and kissing. He added

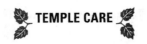

he had also never heard contemporary hymns in church before. He said he began to tap his foot. He asked, "By the way, what race is the pastor?" I told him he was from South Africa: he's African. His expression of joy did not change. I invited he and his wife to the church dedication services.

Our church and our sister church have many people who are obese and/or morbidly obese. I came to see them as embodiments of a growing cultural concern for this issue. The church potluck dinners are like dining at your local all-you-can-eat restaurants and we eat like it is. We sit, eat and fellowship. We have unspoken food contests by simply designating who is to bring certain dishes. The servers set their portions aside to make sure a particular dish has not been consumed before we have finished serving. The members are gaining more and more weight.

I thought about obesity in the church and was impressed to give a message titled Temple Care, using the Biblical image of the body as temple. To be honest, I had to pray against the spirit of fear to give the message; the discussion of obesity (being overweight, "fat") was new. I read Jeremiah 1:7 and 17 and forced myself to give it. It was well-received, and Rev. Hoffman asked me to deliver the same message to our sister church, where a large percentage of the members are morbidly obese. It was the message given at our sister church that ignited the passion to reach out to the obese and morbidly obese in our community, and to engage in critical Scriptural-theological thought about this growing public issue as a chaplain, nurse and Christian woman.

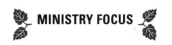
Synergy

As I was researching the Internet for the BMI Chart (which gives proper or ideal weight for one's height and bone structure), I ran across the obesity stats for America. At that time, Indiana was no. 3 on the map according to the Centers for Disease Control. The sermon was altered to fit the need of that particular congregation.

When I walked into the church and saw the size of a large percentage of the people, my heart sank. I said to myself "I see why pastor wanted me to give this message!" I joined in singing praise with the congregation again to block the spirit of fear. The pastor and his wife are slim, fit and excellent examples in every way as Rev. Hoffman is, but I was deeply sensitive to the feelings of the obese.

When I gave the title of the message and my Scripture texts, I then gave the credentials that qualified me to teach a message on *Temple Care,* that of having suffered the physical and psychological pain of being an overweight teen. I then sensed acceptance. It was as though they exhaled.

When I began to teach, a glory cloud (metaphorically speaking of the peace and stillness of God that physically appears foggy), fell over the room. They not only received it, they were like sponges. One of the nurses in the church took the baton to help launch a program on *Temple Care.* Overweight people need help just as drug addicts do; however, they seldom talk about it, being "invisible" and deeply personal. The message spoke to stress, rest and diet, because they all can be connected to weight gain.

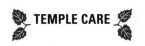

This led to the exploration of Christian and secular resources to approach cultural issues and unrecognized groups of persons needing care. It began with the Creator's action regarding the human being as a spirit, soul, body, chemical, biological, social and one's theological anthropology who humans are as God created us. One's body is as important as one's spirit and soul. As I minister to the obese and morbidly obese in the hospital, when I am impressed to share the pain of having been an overweight teen, the door opens. I then invite that person to join the church congregation for the 21-day workshop that is in the developmental stages as an interdisciplinary program, with the transformative process of Temple Care.

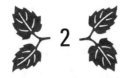

MINISTRY MODEL

Church is home away from home for the Christian family to grow in relationship with God, commune and support each other. For best results, the Creator should be allowed to also navigate the choosing of that house of God. Michael F. Trainer, author of *The Quest for Home*, speaks to the importance of selecting one's church family, because, "There in solitude we recognize our deepest connection with other human beings. The sense of ourselves as religious is enhanced when this social dimension is honored in the Christian setting."[1]

Although we are part of the entire body of Christ, there is a particular community where one can bond, grow spiritually and build relationships with comfort. We are family, brothers and sisters in the Lord. Blood is not thicker than water, spirit is (Mark 3:31-35).

The ecclesia is based on the soteriological work of Jesus Christ. Without a basic understanding of the role Jesus plays in the church, it may become merely a social club. Tyrone Inbody, author of *The Faith of the Christian Church*, says,

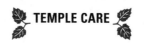

"Christ is more than the church; our relationship to the church is dependent on the church's relation to Christ."[2] The church that has a dependency on Christ, flows with Christ by the leading of the Holy Spirit, therefore, usually thrives.

Each church body is considered a culture. Nancy T. Ammerman says, "All cultures have rituals that give shape to people's common life together, and congregations are certainly no exception."[3] For example, most denominations have a particular order of service they are legalistic about maintaining. However, with some churches, although there is formality for order; leadership yields to the prompting of the Holy Spirit, thus allowing the Holy Spirit to interrupt that pattern according to His Will.

Another ritualistic behavior is the fellowship meal. Potluck meals reflect the many cultures of which River of Life Church is composed: African, African American, Caucasian and Spanish. The food is very tasty and fattening. There is an unspoken contest among the cooks. When meals are planned, certain ones are asked to prepare a particular dish. Therefore, it is known in advance if anyone new brings a dish, it is usually eaten last or left unless someone attests to the tastiness of the food. Healthy, low-fat meals must be encouraged in the churches as examples of the directions given in the Bible and of what has been scientifically proven the best nourishment for humanity.

Rev. Hoffman spoke of some in the church as being spiritually emaciated. He even went on to say we do not have an "upper" room; we have a "supper" room. It appears too much attention is placed on fellowship meals. I have

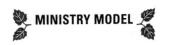

become concerned as I observed many in the congregation as they gained weight and acquired various obesity related diseases. The church must lead by example in every area, including community meals that reflect health and healing and maintenance.

I was successful in locating a wealth of programs encouraging a lifestyle diet the way God designed for His humanity. However, most did not cite that God is the originator of those same scientific directions. God designed the human machine to be fueled and energized by the food substances He has designated in His word, our guidebook, the Bible. The Bible is like any other manual; it remains the same because the model (humanity) has not changed. Through relationship with God, one is directed to apply the contents of the Bible from a contemporary perspective. Walter Brueggemann in his book *The Bible Makes Sense* speaks to this subject from one's ability to visualize, to also be creative. He writes:

> Imagination is the gift of vitality that enables the believing community to discern possibility and promise, to receive newness and healing where others only measure and analyze. From generation to generation, the transmission of the Bible in all its power and vitality has been possible because people with imagination have been sensitive to fresh dimensions of meaning, to new interconnections perceived for the first time, to new glimpses of holiness that lie within the text.[4]

What Brueggemann calls imagination, I call the Spirit of God being developed through that relationship.

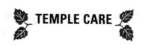

I bring to this project 40 years of knowledge in the medical field as a registered nurse, of which behavioral medicine and addiction treatment units were segments of that experience. In addition, skills acquired along my personal journey to maintain health are incorporated into this discussion for the benefit of others.

The state of the art for this ministry model is the development of the relationship of Temple Care to Improved Health for individuals afflicted with obesity at River of Life Church and the nearby community hospital. This project is built upon the Pastoral Care and Counseling pattern. The pastors lead by example along with other leaders in the church based on God's Word, with scientific underpinning to replace the unhealthy eating habits with those which are nourishing. Stress plays a significant role in most addictions; therefore, it will be addressed. Ample rest is equally vital when losing weight along with proper diet.

Samuel D. Proctor, author of *We Have This Ministry,* defines the role of the pastor as counselor. He writes,

> Ambiguous as the role of counselor may be, a pastor who knows Jesus, who has walked with the Master up and down the dusty roads of Judea, Galilee, Perea, and Samaria, who has accepted Christ as the paradigm of the good life, and who measures his or her own successes and failures by the standards that Jesus set, brings something special to the counseling session. A pastor whose own life has been held together by God's grace, who has found access to the inexhaustible power of God through an unfeigned faith in Jesus as God's self-disclosure in time and space, is enabled to help in ways that are simply unavailable to those who

are strangers to Christ. Such a pastor is at home with brokenness because as God's servant, he or she has dealt with brokenness at close range over and over again. In pursuit of the Jesus paradigm, such a pastor has paid more attention to the fragmented lives than to the ones that are whole. No one can play God, but good pastors are God's instruments and are enabled to help God's people to find wholeness and fulfillment with the finite "stuff" of life.[5]

What Proctor is saying is that, as a counselor and one who has walked the same path as the counselee and felt similar pain, I can therefore direct that person out as Jesus did the counselor. The Biblical counselors on the Temple Care team will be those who have won the battle with obesity.

A listening presence is imperative in the counseling process. In *Hearing Beyond the Words,* Emma J. Justes defines several types or styles of listening. One particular definition that caught my attention regarding the counseling process is listening as Christian Hospitality. She writes, "Hospitality is done with quietness and humility. Humility is in the recognition that what I have to offer is limited, and I recognize that even as a generous host I do not have everything that my guest might need—or everything I need myself."[6] Recognizing one's limitations keeps us dependent on God for both the client and ourselves.

Along with presence and listening, care is very much a part of that pastoral process. That concern requires an individual plan and usually some type of preparation in advance, which may require instruction. Peggy Way, in her book *Created by God,* spoke to that aforethought:

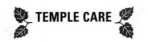

. . . education being a mode of care both because of the close relationship between theories and practices of Christian Education and Pastoral Care, and because educational practices must prepare care-givers and receivers to see need, view themselves as resources, and understand context, and have an intentional grounding in faithfulness.[7]

Dr. Way's statement is a reminder to one who is a pastoral caregiver and receiver that continuing education is imperative as the various needs change. It also says that, although the process of reaching one may be amended, the faith for it to be accomplished remains constant.

I attended a seminar on October 26, 2007, to receive information on how to reach those addicts who do not want help or who are in some form of denial. Those who are addicted to food may fall under one of the above. I was seeking and found a loving way of approaching the loved ones to the obese before they hit rock bottom. Bottom for the drug or alcohol abuser could be a stroke, heart attack and death (to self or others by driving). Ironically, the same can occur with ones who abuse food as a consequence of one or another chronic disease that is a result of obesity.

Jeff Jay and Debra Jay, authors of *Love First* and Professional Interventionists, say that, ". . . its [hitting bottom] the most unchallenged myth about addiction and the one that stops us from responding to a deadly and destructive disease. It leaves us standing at the sidelines while addiction runs through our families like a freight train."[8]

Food addiction, as any other, can be from a family situation, however, not necessarily from genetics. More often

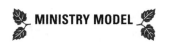

than not, it is from generations of improper eating and/or stress related where food becomes the soother. In the forward to the Jay's book, George McGovern writes, "Intervention is a way of erecting a 'bottom' before such a tragedy occurs."[9] The tragedy that he spoke of was the death of his daughter to alcohol.

The interventionists use love, sometimes very tough love. "It organizes love and honesty and uses them to break through the barriers of addiction."[10] We were manufactured by God's love and therefore can be healed by it from any aspect of sickness. Addiction is beyond human ability; it is conquered by the grace of God (the Christian's higher power).

This technique was discovered when,

> A minister in the 1960s, Dr. Vernon Johnson, and his congregation developed a way families could intervene on an addicted loved one. The intervention techniques were designed for families to use and were not a part of the professional world. Since that time, a new profession has sprung up based on Dr. Johnson's work—The Interventionist.[11]

The Jays go on to define food addicts and mention very important aspects that must be confronted for healing to manifest. They say, "Compulsive overeaters lose control over the amount of food they eat and suffer from obesity . . . Overeating is often related to complicated emotional problems, fear, emotional pain and stress."[12]

Theodore S. Baroody in *Alkalize or Die* defines stress down to the cellular level. What happens when the "fight or take flight" feeling occurs? He says tension occurs,

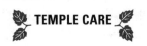

When the system is placed in a fighting posture with no adversary present, excessive hormones are generated causing contraction of muscles and a redirection of digestive forces. Therefore, even alkaline forming foods become acidic. Improper metabolism in the cell forms acid that is not eliminated quickly enough, lessening oxygen intake into the cell causing cellular breakdown, blood and lymph flows are altered. As a consequence, oxygen and nutrients are not carried to the cells nor taken away at the rate they should be. Lymphatic system accumulation then becomes inevitable. These acids create stresses we actually feel.[13]

The Creator did not design the human body to hold the stress and/or toil that came with the fall of humanity (Gen. 3:17). God is to vindicate any situation that may cause stress. The Word says "to be anxious for nothing . . . " (Phil. 4:6). The reason is two-fold: one is spiritual and the other is physical. Do not give place to Satan (Eph. 4:26), and physical stress shuts our immune system down. Stress only causes harm (Ps. 37:8). *Poneras* is a Greek word for harm. *Vine's Bible Dictionary* defines it as, "evil (it denotes what is destructive, injurious), generally of a more malignant sort."[14] *Encarta World Dictionary* defines malignant as, "wanting to do evil, harmful and likely to grow and spread."[15] According to Baroody, for best health, the body should maintain an "80% alkaline reserve and 20% from the acid-forming list."[16] According to his thinking, "Too much acidity in the body is like having too little oil in your car. It just grinds to a halt one lazy Sunday afternoon."[17]

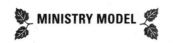

Laughter is said to create an alkaline physiological state. "A merry heart doth good, like medicine, but a broken spirit dries the bones" (Prov. 17:22). Immune Systems Health Information is in accord with Baroody. It affirms that,

> Your immune system function can be compromised by stress, anger, anxiety, depression, envy, hostility or resentment. Each emotion can suppress your immune system in minutes and last for hours. Within fifteen minutes of a stressful situation our immune system is so severely suppressed that it may fail to mount the counter attack against the enemy. Our stressful lifestyles, jobs and relationships can leave us vulnerable to issues such as cancer cells, infection or allergies to name a few.[18]

Resting the body is important, especially for one who is obese and trying to lose weight. According to Baroody, a lack of rest also renders the system acidic. He says,

> Sleep is a sense, and as such is as important to life as seeing, tasting, smelling and hearing. During the sleep period, many acid by-products brought about by over-exhaustion, are processed and eliminated from the body through deep breathing and sweating. This repair period is alkaline producing in nature.[19]

Scientists all over the United States and abroad are talking about the connection between obesity, lack of sleep and apnea problems for adults, as well as children. Patricia Neighmond published the results of two related topics.

> Two studies report that sleep loss can contribute to obesity. Researchers found that when men slept 10 hours, they awoke with normal appetites. But

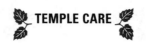
when they slept only four hours they were hungry. And what they wanted to eat wasn't lean meats, fruits or vegetables.[20]

Neal Barnard adds to that, saying,

Exercise is like a giant reset button on your body. When you have a good workout several vitally important things happen; it blocks appetite swings, it resets your mood, and your exercise-rest cycle so you can sleep properly-which strengthens you against cravings; and it puts you in a different relationship with your body.[21]

I am also encouraging the various pastors to set up workout rooms in the churches. With the pastor's lead, it will hopefully encourage congregants to follow. Rev. Ron Gaston is an assistant pastor at New Hope Missionary Baptist Church in Michigan City, IN, as well as a certified fitness professional. He has combined the two by creating the Temple Total Fitness Program for kids, 10-15. He is conducting a 12-week pilot program for 28 kids whose body mass index (BMI) puts them in the overweight or obese category. They are also making a connection between what they eat and drink and how they feel about themselves 219-448-0719.

Michigan City schools wellness policy:

Michigan City Area School Board recognizes that good nutrition and regular physical activity affect the health and well-being of the corporation's students . . . furthermore with objectives of enhancing student health and well-being, and reducing childhood obesity, the following policy: Policy number 8510 and others contained more information than space

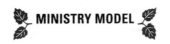

allows. Goal I: Nutrition will be further; integrated into all areas of the curriculum whenever possible . . . Goal II: Nutrition education will involve sharing information with families and the broader community. (www.mcas.k12.in.us/admin.asp?page=supmes)

Professor Cappuccio defines scientific reasoning further for clarity. He points out that "Short sleep duration may lead to obesity through an increased appetite via hormonal changes caused by the sleep deprivation. Lack of sleep produces Ghrelin, among other effects, stimulates appetite and creates less Leptin which, among other effects, suppresses appetite . . ."[22]

He went on to give that sleeplessness a name; he called it a "silent epidemic."[23] Most adults, teens and children in today's society do not get ample rest for one reason or another. Rest and sleep are important contributing factors to health, maintenance and longevity which one must put forth a conscious effort to accomplish. As previously stated, eight hours is needed to rebuild and repair cells.

The more weight one gains creates further problems with sleeping, such as apnea, which is "temporary absence of breathing."[24] In a study conducted by Krista L. Haines and several others, it was reported "obstructive sleep apnea (OSA) is associated with obesity."[25] It appears our bodies were not designed to hold stress and not have ample rest. God seems to have programmed us to depend on Him by choice to vindicate our situations (Rom. 12:19). We may need to add a prayer for sweet sleep (Prov. 3:24), and that is okay because the Word says, "Pray without ceasing" (1 Thess. 5:17).

Experts also say proper exercise and diet are equally as important as sleep. However, something as simple as walking can be painful for one who is carrying an extra 50 or 100 pounds. Sadly, the obese/morbidly obese move as little as possible. Water Aerobics is the best way to get them moving and have fun while doing so. Exercise raises one's heart rate and in doing so pumps the blood faster, thereby pushing cholesterol out of the arteries, increasing circulation and healing. Charles Emery, a professor at Ohio State University, found that "regular exercise can boost the healing process by as much as 25 percent, according to a fascinating study . . ."[26] The article went on to explain that "exercise increases circulation and helps regulate the immune system and hormones that influence the healing process."[27]

Dr. Leland Winston wrote the forward for Martha White's book titled, *Water Exercises,* speaking to its benefits. He attests that "water therapy is an excellent method to use when normal gravity conditions might make the rehabilitation process painful and even dangerous."[28] White says water exercise is easier on the body. She documents that "due to the decrease of gravitational forces in the water, the body moves freely and the overall weight is diminished so that a body part, such as a leg, can be lifted and stretched without as much pain."[29] I have experienced the comfort of water aerobics and therefore have incorporated it into the Temple Care Workshop. Many have described the after feeling as that of having had a massage.

An article written in "Diabetic Lifestyle" recommends water aerobics as an exercise. The article also explains how the water makes it easier on one's body than floor exercise.

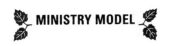

"The buoyancy supports your body so that you can protect your joints, muscles and bones. Remember that at chest level, you will have 85%-90% of your body supported."[30]

Up to this point, I have narrated some of the aspects of Temple Care, which are: Biblical Pastoral Counseling, care, listening, stress, rest and water aerobics. The pastoral counselor should be one who has won the battle with obesity for best results. One special skill the counselor should have is listening. Listening as hospitality was discussed. Care was spoken of from the perspective to educating oneself regarding self-care. Water aerobics was defined because it is one of the best forms of exercise for one who is obese. Proper diet is imperative for health and maintenance, along with drinking good water and all of the above. Included will be some of the similar programs that are having success such as; eating an abundance of fruit and vegetables.

Some people, due to a disability or use of a wheelchair, cannot exercise as freely. Light weight-bearing exercise is excellent to maintain strength in the arms and shoulders.

Disabilities should not deter people from attaining the positive benefits of a well-structured weight program. Strength training increases muscle size, improves muscle endurance, prevents bone loss and increases self-esteem. Weight training will not only make a person stronger, it can also ward off common injuries to areas such as the shoulders and elbows. More importantly, people with disabilities should partake in weight training activities to the extent their abilities allow to prevent loss of function or autonomy.[31]

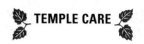

The American Association on Health and Disability (AAHD) promotes and supports wellness. People with disabilities may have to be more careful to reduce the incidents of secondary conditions, such as the named diseases as a result of inactivity and improper diet.

I recommend a machine called the Theracycle 200. It is a motor-powered, computer-monitored fitness machine designed to guide the user through a programmed workout in the home. The machine looks similar to a bicycle. You sit on the seat, strap in the feet and hands, turn it on to a specified workout and the machine does it. Everyone needs some form of exercise.

Dr. Terry Mason, Chicago commissioner of health, agrees that "a diet rich in fruits and vegetables as part of an active lifestyle lowers the risk of every diet related disease."[32] He introduced a program that is most closely associated with Temple Care at the United Theological Seminary's January Intensive of 2006. The program is called "Body and Soul." Dr. Mason spoke to the role of the church in health, posing the questions: "How many of you have members of your church that have high blood pressure, diabetes, heart trouble, overweight, cancer? How about family and friends?"[33] Dr. Mason went on to document that "African Americans suffer disproportionately from many major health problems."[34] The above questions can be addressed by a congregational nurse in an effort to provide holistic care from the church perspective along the line of prevention. This program has also incorporated two related scriptures, Gen. 1:29 expresses the original diet of fruit and 1Cor. 6:19 speaks to the body of the

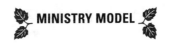

individual Christian as "a temple of the Holy Spirit." Dr. Mason explains that,

> Body and Soul is a wellness program for African-American churches. It empowers church members to eat more fruits and vegetables for better health. The program was developed by the National Cancer Institute in collaboration with The American Cancer Society, the University of North Carolina, and University of Michigan.[35]

The African American is also the minority obese in America where obesity is epidemic. That says to me other cultures are facing the same issue on a grand scale around the globe. Nonetheless, the African American is at high risk of the above named diseases as a result of a high fat diet that has been passed on from generation to generation (see slave diet in the history chapter).

Of Faith and Food is another interesting nutritional program also aimed at African-American churches. The project is called,

> The PRAISE! (Partnership to Reach African-Americans to Increase Smart Eating!) Project, with its 60 partici-pating churches in eight North Carolina counties, began with a call from the National Cancer Institute (NCI) for nutrition interventions (programs that help make behavior changes), aimed at minorities.[36]

This study also addressed the high-fat meat some African Americans consume. It was conducted by the University of North Carolina's Research Department.

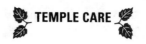

Bethany Jackson, Clinical Associate Professor of Nutrition, emphasized the healthful components present in the population's diet and suggested ways to modify traditional recipes to meet NCI's, dietary guidelines without sacrificing taste. . . . For example, collards, a great choice nutritionally, became a high-fat, high-salt food when seasoned with ham hocks or fat back. PRAISE! suggested using chicken broth and smoked turkey instead.[37]

Again, the NCI recognized that in any study there are obstructions to overcome before it can proceed. "Among the [barriers to recruiting churches] were credibility, trust, tradition and economics, says Lee Downing, pastor of Friendship Missionary Baptist church in Fayetteville, NC."[38] Past injuries to a culture can cause such hindrances. Trust was a definite issue in this situation that had to be addressed.

Many congregants knew about the infamous Tuskegee Syphilis Study (1932-1972), in which researchers withheld treatment from 400 black men without their informed consent. The PRAISE! Team addressed concerns by discussing Tuskegee openly and vowing to share fully all information from the study. President Clinton's formal apology for Tuskegee May 1997 increased concern. Four attorneys who were members of a participating church, unsettled by the potential for DNA testing, grilled one staff member on the specifics of blood collection. The team revised the PRAISE! consent form stipulation that blood samples would be used only for nutrition-related measures . . .[39]

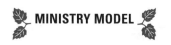

Once trust has been breeched, it is difficult to believe. This group had "Joseph Paige, former dean of the Shaw University School of Divinity. He provided Biblical references so pastors could incorporate the project into their services. Citing 1 Cor. 3:16 Paige suggested stressing that the human body is God's temple, and that to do God's work an individual must be healthy."[40] The Scripture cited is speaking to the body of Christ corporately. The PRAISE! program turns out to be another success story proven by research scientists that a diet abundant in fruits and vegetables is best for humanity.

There are pastors who preach and live segments of the Word. The areas they are in rebellion against are usually not spoken to. Some of those pastors are included in the over-weight/obese/morbidly obese categories. They preach about drug addiction and alcohol and never touch food addiction (gluttony). One article caught my attention that spoke to inactivity, which mentioned that reading the Bible is seden-tary, talking about fat preachers. The article answered by saying, "It is not the reading of the Bible which causes obesity—and other failures . . . it is the failure to Understand and Obey the Bible which is the problem."[41] We must lead by example in all areas of the Word. We must admit our short-comings as leaders for the others to realize that through Christ, any failing can be reversed.

It is not only the overeating that contributes to the obesity; it is some of the additives, according to Kevin Trudeau, author of *Natural Cures,*

> Fat people eat more food. Chemicals are being added to our food that actually makes us gain weight. The

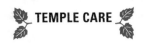

more fat people there are, the more profits there are for the food industry. The most shocking part of this is one such chemical put in most "diet food." How sad that an unknowing consumer buys some food that has the word "diet" on it in hopes of losing some weight, when actually eating the food causes them to gain weight.[42]

Trudeau is encouraging the public to revert to natural food as much as possible. He continues to disclose the deceit of a particular manufacturer as an example.

Food manufacturers are knowingly putting chemicals into food that cause the consumer to become physically addicted to it. We know that drugs, which are chemicals, can be incredibly physically and emotionally addictive. . . . In the book *The Real Thing: The truth and power at the Coca Cola company,* the story of how cocaine was an important ingredient in Coca-Cola is exposed. One of the main reasons cocaine was such an important ingredient was that the consumer unknowingly became addicted to Coca-Cola. Having a person addicted to your product is good for your profits . . .[43]

I was a young girl during the Coca-Cola scandal. As children, we were not allowed to drink it, nor coffee. We must continue to screen and read labels as much as possible. In today's society, even if the label says organic, is it really? Trudeau says, "Virtually everything that you put into your mouth has pesticides, herbicides, antibiotics, growth hormone, genetically altered material or food additives."[44] The above certainly attests to the fact that there are many factors that contribute to obesity that are not under one's

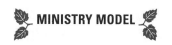

control. However, as consumers, one can choose the most natural products and learn to read labels. Someone said, "If you can't pronounce it, don't eat it." Sneed cites information that will aid in the label reading of beef.

> The Environmental Newsletter (May 1992) pointedly asks if the substance we often make into meat loaf should be more correctly called ground beef or ground fat. This is a question of significance, since beef makes up to 44 percent of the total meat sales in the U.S., causing it to be the single largest source of fat in the American diet.[45]

We not only need to read, we must also learn to translate codes and labeling language.

Labeling on ground beef is expressed as % lean by weight. But thinking of it in terms of % calories from fat is more revealing.

Ground Beef labeled as	Provides
73% lean	79% percent calories from fat
80% lean	71% percent calories from fat
85% lean	64% percent calories from fat
90% lean	53% percent calories from fat
95% lean	34% percent calories from fat[46]

Labeling, along with ingredients, has not been totally honest in many situations. It would be wise to take a consumer class or seminar on labeling. Even something that has been deemed in the Bible as a meat source has been polluted by industry. There again, is why choice comes in to play. We must choose where and what we purchase. We may

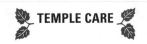

have to travel to purchase the best meat; nonetheless, it is worth it.

"Pork is the highest among all meat at 91% fat."[47] It is also said to be a carrier of flu viruses and various worms. Just think, one could get the flu from eating a bacon, lettuce and tomato or ham sandwich, and wonder where the flu bug came from. ". . . The immune system of pigs is similar to that of humans and the animals suffer from a wide variety of diseases that also infect people. Scientists say the bird flu pathogen would swap genes with a human influenza virus inside a pig."[48]

Flood goes on to say, "It should also be pointed out that influenza epidemics are virtually unheard of in the Muslim countries, where pork is not eaten."[49] That certainly is good news. I have never had a flu shot or the flu and have not eaten pork since 1972.

High fat content and the flu virus are not the only things that are harmful (malignant) about the pig. Flood found,

> The trichina is not just one worm found in the swine. There is a large round worm, the gullet worm, three kinds of stomach worm, a tiny hairworm, a hookworm, and the thorn headed worm in the small intestine. There are several species of nodular worms and one species of whipworm in the large intestines, and the kidney worm. The large round worm can be as big as eighteen inches.[50]

Could the above be the "abomination that the Word is speaking of?" Perhaps the oozing of the worms through the skin of the swine, as one pig owner expressed to me, is

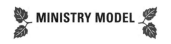

another reason we are not even to touch them? Our bodies can be built up or broken down from the food we eat.

A nutritionist from Jewel Food stores, speaking on Channel 7 TV news, mentioned seven foods we should not live without that boost energy and increase sleep. She explained,

That an *apple* a day fights cancer and cholesterol, and *citrus* fruit all colors, *olive* oil is also good for arthritis. *Greens* are good for vision and memory. *Strawberries* boost memory and immune system. *Grapes* are good for heart health, BP, Ca (dark colors), and *walnuts* have melatonin which boosts sleep. She encourages sprinkling a few on your salad. [emphasis added][51]

She agrees that raw fruits and vegetables are medicine.

I have attested to the healing properties in carrots in my spiritual autobiography. Jean Carper, author of *The Food Pharmacy,* speaks to the healing properties in carrots. She says,

The essence of carrot has already been widely tested in humans as a potential antidote to cancer. Although every food in a grab bag of chemicals that attack cancer broadly, the carrot factor, it appears, interferes with the cancer process at later stages-during the promotion phase. And its orangeness may perform best against cancers peculiarly related to smoking.[52]

Again, this is God's natural medicine from His garden.

I was given an article from a men's magazine that featured a story of a 38-year-old man wanting to cleanse his body of toxins. What caught my eye was that the person the article referenced spoke of God as if knowing the proper diet; however, he chose what tasted good until negative changes

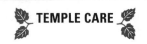

in his body were observed. At that point, he was not interested in a quick fix; he knew it had to be a lifestyle change. I could sense his exhaustion when he said, "I wanted to look into a plate of raw veggies and see God."[53]

That said to me he understood the connection between a relationship with God through a healthy temple with the food God specifically designed for the purpose of health and maintenance.

Some people live to eat; therefore, they usually have improper diets that lead to obesity and health issues related to being obese. The created must eat food that was specifically designed by the Creator, not chemical foodstuffs made by the creation. "The whole point of eating is to maintain and promote bodily health. Hippocrates' famous injunction to let food be thy medicine is ritually invoked to support this notion."[54]

There is food we can eat that will protect, and other chemically manufactured substances, when eaten, will leave the body vulnerable for invasion by cancer and other abnormal cells. "Researchers have long believed based on epidemiological comparisons of different populations, that diet high in fruits and vegetables confers some protection against cancer."[55] The aforementioned about raw carrot juice is an example. On the third day, God created the food source for His humanity which was ". . . the herb that yields seed, and the fruit tree that yields fruit according to its kind (Genesis 1:9-12). Then He created humanity in this self-contained environment. There were no doctors then, therefore the healing properties in the herbs and fruit were

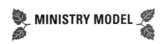

established by God before doctors or scientists came into existence. Some scientists believe they have discovered the healing properties in fruits and vegetables; however, it was already innately there.

The following chapter will speak to the Biblical stance of the Creator's plan of care for His creation from a holistic perspective: spirit, soul and body. The focus will be on God's original diet plan for His creation, which is the same yesterday, today and forever.

3

BIBLICAL FOUNDATION

In the beginning, God methodically created a perfect habitat for His creation to have dominion, to cohabit with the environment and thrive therein—the Garden of Eden. According to DNA study, the garden is located in the Mediterranean, where the origin of humanity was traced. "A recent African origin of modern humans, although still disputed, is supported now by a majority of genetic studies."[1] Genesis 2:10-14 is the Biblical source that speaks to the garden location. With the human design and creation, later came the manual for upkeep and longevity of life for the whole person (spirit, soul and body). The Bible is "The canonical writings accepted as normal for a religious faith. In Christianity, the Old Testament (Hebrew Scriptures) and the New Testament comprise the Bible. Theologically, the Bible is acknowledged in the church as revelation from God."[2] The specialty of the Bible is to "function as providing a source and norm for such elements as belief, conduct, and experience of God."[3]

The Bible is my guidebook and I have faith that "all scripture is given by inspiration of God, and is profitable for

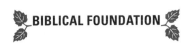
reproof, for correction, for instruction in righteousness" (2 Tim. 3:16).[4] Migliore gives clarity to the same scripture from a contemporary perspective. He says, "Basically, the doctrine affirms that God the Holy Spirit accompanied and guided the human writers of the scripture, respecting their humanity in all limitations and its conditioning by historical, social and cultural context, yet conveying God's Word through the human witnesses."[5] Among authors in pastoral care literature, there is a general understanding of the spiritual, social-cultural, moral and biological-chemical wholeness of the human creature.

Anyone who drives an automobile will follow their manual, as it is written by the manufacturer for the best life and longevity of the vehicle, no matter how ancient it becomes. I suggest humanity should have no less respect for its own personal manual, the Bible.

America is bordering on a pandemic of obesity, according to the Center for Disease Control. Citizens have consulted many other diet books and followed their laws (system of rules), and it appears to have failed more often than not. I am simply suggesting humanity try its own guidebook for best results. The old saying goes, "If all else fails, follow the directions." A good example is putting together a bicycle without reading or following the directions, and when it's all assembled discovering there are screws left in the plastic bag that are not considered extra according to the instructions. This argument states my core biblical hermeneutic, as well as calls for a dialogue between the Bible and, as nurse/chaplain, the social, scientific and biochemical understanding of the human.

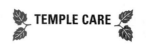

The focus of this Biblical exploration will be on spirit, soul and body, concentrating on the care of one's body (Temple) from a scriptural perspective. Care is primary to this study; therefore, it will be defined for that purpose. It is equally important for the reader to understand why I address the body as the temple. There are four scriptures I use for the understanding and underpinning of this research project. They are: Gen. 1:29-30; Gen. 9:2-3; Lev. 11:1-8 and 1 Cor. 6:19-20. This area will conclude with five particular scriptures I have selected to explain that God has not changed regarding the food laws as some understand it to be, because of one or the other said scriptures.

Spirit, Soul and Body

Humanity is also triune in the image of God. I further have faith that I am a spirit (the breath of life that came from God, which gave life and animation), and that I possess a soul (the mind, intellect, will and emotion), and I dwell in a body (the earth suit or one's temple).

Many use spirit and soul interchangeably. Spirit and soul are different, yet the same, implying they are both spirit. Romans 8:27 speaks to one's spirit mind, which is housed in one's physical brain. Just as one's spirit mind resides in one's physical brain, one's spirit body dwells within one's physical body. At death, one's spirit and soul go as a unit to be with the Lord for the balance of eternity, while one's physical body and head are buried as a unit and go back to the dust they were created from (Gen. 3:19; Luke 16:19-31). *Vine's Bible Dictionary* says, "apparently, then the relationship may be

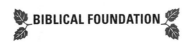

summed up *soma,* body, and *pneuma,* spirit, may be separated [at death], *pneuma,* and *psuche,* can only be distinguished."[6] This quote says to me that although *pneuma* (spirit) and *psuche* (mind) are both spirit, they can be recognized as different.

It has been my experience and tradition that the spirit mind is that part of the human that makes the decisions or choice to live for God or one's body which cannot be renewed. My understanding is that this is the reason why, when one is born anew, one's mind must be renewed by the Word of God, reprogrammed so to speak.

McKim speaks to spirit, soul and body from another perspective. He says:

> The spirit (*pneuma*) is a being that does not have a material substance. This includes God (John 4:24), The Holy Spirit as the third person of the Trinity [Godhead] and the dimension of human life that enables a relationship with God.[7]

McKim goes on to say,

> The creationist point of view of soul is that God directly created a new "soul" at the instant of one's conception. This would mean that the soul is not transmitted naturally by the parents . . . Mortal body (*soma*) the present, physical body of a person which is susceptible to death and theologically the power of sin.[8]

This understanding grounds my belief in the wholeness of God's creation of persons (human beings).

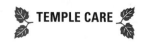

Care

Care is intentional and necessary for the survival of the person. There are many types and definitions of care; however, for the purpose of this study, the goal is body (temple) care. *Vine's Bible Dictionary* says, "Care involves direction of the mind toward the object cared for."[9] Self care is also not any one single thing usually. Although instructions for humanity's diet are listed in the Bible, other scientific knowledge is needed primarily for understanding the Creator's dietary regulations for best health from a contemporary perspective.

Dr. Peggy Way addressed in her book *Created by God* some of the many aspects of Care:

> First, care is a human not a professional function. For the human care is a biological imperative, intrinsic in the creation of the human infant as helpless as needing physical and emotional caring practices to survive.[10]

I will tag onto that statement "and to thrive." This quote also reminds me of the fact that self-sufficient adults will also always need help with that self-care from others. Help in the sense of understanding and direction regarding what foods physically support the body to function at its optimum and what foods that could be detrimental to one's health. Dr. Way also speaks to that intentional focus. She says,

> . . . education being a mode of care both because of the close relationship between theories and practices of Christian education and pastoral care, and because educational practices must prepare caregivers and

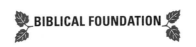

receivers to see need, view themselves as resource, and understand context, and have an intentional grounding and foundation in faithfulness.[11]

Dr. Way's above quote reminds me we are all primary care-givers and receivers to ourselves, as well as to others. One cannot simply become hearers of the Word; one has to also become a doer of the Word, put theory into practice. God desires for us to prosper and be in health, even as our soul prospers (3 John 2), so that God can navigate the body toward what God has ordained for us to do/and be for others as pastoral caregivers.

Tabernacle/Temple

The Tabernacle constructed by Moses in the wilderness was the model or blueprint for the temples that were built thereafter by Solomon, Zerrubbabel and Herod, on earth patterned after the heavenly original. God said to Moses, "According to all that I show you, that is the pattern of the tabernacle and the pattern of all of its furnishings, just so you shall make it" (Ex. 25:9). There were exact dimensions, only certain woods, metals, animal skins and clothing that were to be used, and those who gave it had to do so from a loving heart. The New Testament also attests to the importance of the directions of the tabernacle being adhered to exactly, and it being a heavenly prototype. "They offer worship in a sanc-tuary that is a sketch and shadow of the heavenly one; for Moses when he was about to erect the tent, he was warned, see that you make everything to the pattern that was shown you on the mountain" (Heb. 8:2-6).

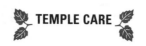

If Moses was disobedient and the pattern was off the slightest degree, would we have missed Jesus? They had faith to obey as a result of the signs and wonders they had experienced along their journey of deliverance. It is important to understand that God has a perfect plan and purpose for everything God says or does for humanity.

The plan of the first tabernacle in the Old Testament wilderness was for it to be a dwelling place for God and a place for the sacrifice of animals for the atonement of their sins. It is a specific place to build relationships with God, although God is omnipresent. God ordained the animal sacrifice as a result of the fall of humanity, the disobedience of Adam and Eve. The animal sacrifice was the foundation of the Creator's plan to reconcile the creation to God (2 Cor. 5:18-21). Many scholars say Adam and Eve's son Abel's sacrifice of the first born of his flock was the first. I argue God Himself paved the way again through example by sacrificing an animal to clothe them both after they sinned and realized they were naked and ashamed (Gen 3:21).

The purpose of using the various metals down to the smallest details was a way of communication through the symbolic meaning they each represent. Each article, piece of furniture and tent covering all directed them to our Lord and Savior, Jesus Christ: see Exodus 25.

Many people do not see or understand the connection between the Old and New Testament and therefore separate the Old as no longer relevant or part of the New. Some in society have never met their great-grandparents; however, there remains a connection, a history that can give understanding to the now. Like the human body, the canon is also a whole document gifting our understanding of our created selves.

On the night Jesus was crucified, he said, "I am able to destroy the Temple of God and to build it in three days," referring of course to the resurrection. He also said "I" meaning He laid down His own life for us willingly, and He also referred to His body as The Temple of God. After the ascension, the bodies of believers became that earthly abode, the Temple of the Holy Spirit as one develops a relationship with the Lord (John 2:19-22).

There were and are those of both Christian and Jewish interpretations who have missed it, who are dying for lack of knowledge regarding Tabernacle/Temple significance. Randall Price, author of *The Temple and Bible Prophecy*, speaks to that situation:

> In Christianity, the understanding of the Temple has largely been a history of misunderstanding. This has been because in general Christians look at the Temple as a part of Jewish history and see no connection with Christianity. Historically, whereas the observant Jew had difficulties with the loss of a Temple, but found a substitute in the Torah study of the Temple rulings, the faithful Christian had difficulty from the beginning with the Temple and its rulings and found replacement for them in the church and its rituals.[12]

In this scenario, there are zealous Jews who are in the evangelistic mode, yet waiting for the Messiah. On the other hand, there are a group of compassionate Christians who are

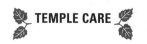

being moved by emotion instead of knowledge desiring to reunite with the Jews. Price documents, "Christian Zionists have, especially for the past decade, embarked upon the road that supports Judaism in the aspiration for a rebuilt Temple."[13] So, each of them has an inadequate understanding of the true significance of the Temple.

A recent article published in Time magazine spoke to the subject of Christian misinterpretation of Tabernacle/Temple. It cites, "Temple restoration is also a fixation for literal-minded Protestants, who deem a new Temple the precondition for Christ's second coming."[14]

There is a serious dilemma within our Christian heritage, that of division of beliefs and styles of worship, governance and interpretations of the Word. The creation has made difficult something the Creator made so simple. Jesus said, "Follow me!" I understand that to mean developing a relationship with Jesus by His direction.

Finally, the Tabernacle/Temple was architecturally designed according to specific dimensions. The Tabernacle/Temple was the center of worship. God's desire is to rebuild His new Temple also according to specifications by His Word. The Christian body, the new Temple, becomes that Holy Sanctuary and present center of worship. I believe God also programmed into each human DNA chain, specific body (Temple) height and weight proportions for ultimate health and longevity. The Creator planted the best maintenance plan before He created and set humanity in the Garden.

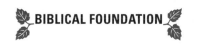

Old Testament

Genesis 1:29-30

And God said, "See I have given you every herb that yields seed which is on the face of the earth, and every tree whose fruit yields seed; to you it shall be for food. Also, to every beast of the earth, to every bird of the air, and to everything that creeps on the earth, in which there is life, I have given every green herb for food, and it was so" (NKJV The Open Bible).

Humankind was originally meant to be fruitarian according to God's Word. It was after the fall when humanity became vegetarian and meat eaters. Man had to work and till the ground for their food. They were locked out of the Garden. Thereafter, they did not have access to the abundance of fruit and medicinal herbs they once had.

One of the words in the Greek language that has several different meanings is "herb." The Greek word "*Lachanon* denotes a garden herb which is a culinary and medicinal plant."[15] Therefore, the "herb" used in Genesis 1:29 was for Adam and Eve's medicinal purposes.

The Creator did not name a particular fruit that was part of their diet which was the cause of the temptation. However, the interpreters chose the red apple which, by the way, is an acid food from the nutritional perspective. According to Theodore A. Baroody, author of *Alkalize or Die,* the yellow golden apple is basic and therefore better. He says the healthy diet consists of "80% basic and 20% acid foods."[16]

I looked up the nutritional value of the apple. It appears to be a complete food, which makes it more understandable why

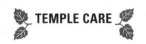

one should eat an "apple a day to keep the doctor away." According to the Australian Custard Apple Growers Association:

> Custard apples provide a well-balanced food source with ample protein, mineral, vitamins, energy and essential fiber. Vitamins A and C are vital for healthy skin, eyes, hair and body tissues. They battle those elements of age and destroy bad cells. Magnesium is nature's tranquilizer. It helps cleanse our systems, improves endurance and our ability to process oxygen and body-building amino acids.[17]

The above quote contains only the nutritional value of the apple. I am sure God had a well-planned fruitarian diet that was not only very filling, but was also tasty. I would imagine Adam and Eve dined on frequent small meals of a variety of healthy, pesticide free, fruit.

I also argue the animals were vegetarian and docile before the fall and assert that "green herb" in verse 30 comes from the Greek word "*fotane,* which denotes grass, fodder or from *basko,* to feed."[18] Animals became carnivores and humans began to eat vegetables. Most animals were ground dwellers, therefore vegetarian and docile, before the fall. Vegetables were also good for humanity before the fall, only man did not have to work to grow them.

The word "herb" addressed in Genesis 3:17-18 is *lachaino* (vegetables). "Lachaino is Greek for herb that means to dig."[19] Humanity did not have to dig until post fall and probably did not understand how the dew watered the garden. It is important to recognize food in creation has a particular role in health, healing and maintenance. The difference in the various cultural settings is mainly in the preparations.

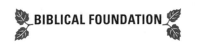
Genesis 9:2-4

The fear and dread of you shall rest on every animal of the earth, and on every bird of the air, on everything that creeps on the ground and on all the fish of the sea; into your hand they are delivered. Every moving thing that lives shall be for food for you; and just as I gave you the green plants, I give you everything. Only you shall not eat flesh with its life, that is, its blood.

The fear and dread God spoke about was for humans to now fear the animals they must hunt if they chose to eat meat. Humanity no longer has dominion over the animals in the same vein as they did in pre-fall days. The animals were no longer orderly and meek; some were very dangerous to humans and were themselves predators looking for meat. Sin had a ripple effect on every living thing. The animals and humans are now in fear of each other. Joseph Blenkinsopp, author of *The Pentateuch, an Introduction to the First Five Books of the Bible,* presents an exegesis that clarifies the point from a different perspective that is relevant for this study. "It is not, however an integral restoration. The permission to eat meat, and therefore to kill, indicates a lower order of existence and the loss of a primordial harmony . . ."[20]

God's method of gradually teaching humanity was through signs and wonders until literacy occurred. It is clear they were given the choice; however, they did not have the benefit of consulting the Bible because they were living through it. God had plans to gradually govern what they should and shouldn't eat beginning in verse 4, which instructs them "not to eat flesh with its life, that is, its blood." That was the beginning of the first laws, the Noachide laws.

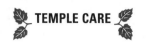

"Briefly stated, these include six proscriptions-against idolatry, bloodshed, blasphemy, theft, sexual sins and eating the flesh of a living animal—and the charge to set up a legal system."[21]

From within this controversial dialogue, John H. Walton speaks to the tolerance for humanity to eat animal flesh. Although I concluded with the same understanding as the author holds, yet he explained the situation differently.

> . . . While meat is not granted for food until after the flood, some have argued that vegetarianism is the ideal and permission to eat meat is only a concession to our fallenness. The first objection against this is that if and when God makes concessions to our fallenness, it is not done by allowing something immoral or sinful in any way, for such concessions would compromise his integrity. The most we may conclude here is that eating meat is not ideal.[22]

This yielding on behalf of our Creator was not compromise; it was a first step in God's plan of redemption for humanity. God also led the way by example. Thus, He sacrificed the first animal to cover the sins of Adam and Eve by also covering their nakedness (Gen. 3:21).

Leviticus 11:1-8

The Lord spoke to Moses and Aaron, saying to them: "Speak to the people of Israel, saying: From the land animals, these are the creatures that you may eat. Any animal that has divided hoofs is cleft footed and chews a cud-such as you may eat. But among those that chew the cud or have divided hoofs, you shall not eat the following: the camel, for even though it chews the cud, it does not have divided hoofs; it is unclean for you. The rock badger, for even though it chews the cud, it does not have divided hoofs; it is unclean for you. The hare, even though it chews the cud, it does not have divided hoofs; it is unclean for you. The pig, for even though it has divided hoofs; and is cleft-footed, it does not chew the cud, it is unclean for you. Of their flesh you shall not eat, and their carcasses you shall not touch; they are unclean for you."

God gave Moses the laws to govern and direct the people toward self-care because they knew not. However, it does not say who penned the Pentateuch. Our Christian foundation is birthed from Jewish tradition, and the Old Testament books have been accepted as canon. There has been much controversy regarding who wrote the first five books of the Bible. "Thus in Spain in the 10th century a certain Ibn Hazam of Cordova, who was really an adherent of the Islamic faith, regarded much of the Pentateuch, including Leviticus as having been compiled by Ezra."[23]

Many have given various perspectives on Moses not being the author; however, most appear to be nonbelievers or opponents of some sort. "Andreas Bodenstein (5th century), an opponent of Martin Luther, maintained Moses could not have possibly composed his own obituary passage in Deuteronomy 34, and argued from the position to a rejection of Moses as the author of the entire Pentateuch, since for him the whole corpus of laws was written in the same broad style as the notice of Moses' death."[24]

Whether the Pentateuch was penned by Moses or someone else translated it from stone, it is widely believed

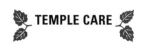

God gave it to Moses. Roy Gane, the author of *Leviticus and Numbers, the NIV Application Commentary* says:

> If you are thinking of the human author, Leviticus consistently maintains that the chief recipient and transmitter of its divine speeches was Moses, so it can be regarded as coauthored. The bibliographic reference could read: God and Moses, Leviticus (Sinai: Israel Publications, second millennium B. C.).[25]

Leviticus teaches excellence in every way. It not only gives instructions in holiness, how to worship and obey a holy God, it also gives direction for personal and public health. As in all ages, humans sought guidance in daily living. We not only worship by rituals and external ceremonies, we are to reverence our bodies (temples) where, in many present day understandings, God presently resides.

Everything that God made was good, for the purpose intended. Anything that is used outside of its created purpose is a perversion. Why are animals classified? Meeks expresses it clearly: "The classification is the result not of empirical medical knowledge, but the universal need to classify phenomena by establishing beneficent and destructive categories."[26] Universal is defined as affecting the whole of humanity, the world.

The Bible says that pig is an abomination, which is according to *Vine's,*

> an object of disgust, something that someone or something as essentially unique in the sense of being dangerous or sinister and repulsive to another individual, characteristics that are detestable to another

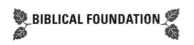

because they are contrary to His nature, things related to death and idolatry, thou shall not eat abominable things (Deut. 14:3), is said of deceivers who profess to know God, but deny Him by their works.[27]

So, if God says a particular food is an abomination, we should pay close attention and not ingest it. Among the prohibited foods are rabbit, swine, catfish, shrimp, lobster tails, whatever crawls on its belly and more. God had a plan and purpose for the dietary laws, and that is to keep His temple healthy and Holy. Even as now, humans seek guidance for what is best for them, and this always includes dialogue with the surrounding cultures.

Thus, contemporary scientists have discovered the animals God forbade humans to consume are the scavenger crew in the animal world, such as swine, shrimp, lobster and catfish. They keep the natural environment clean. "They feed on dead and rotting flesh and discarded scraps."[28] Swine are noted to eat their own dead offspring. They can eat poisonous snakes and, in a matter of hours, it is meat on their bones. It is their nature, what they were created for, and they are good for their created purpose.

The Levitical food laws are identical to those in the Torah. Some people that lack biblical/scientific knowledge may think the pig is dirty or "unclean" because it likes mud and all it needs is a good bath before slaughter. Unclean in what way needs to be clarified. *Eerdmans Commentary* on Leviticus says:

Clean animals must chew the cud and have cloven hoofs. One without the other makes the animal

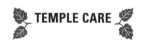
unclean. The pig is unclean because it only has half of the necessary qualifications, divided hoofs, but it does not chew the cud.[29]

That is not enough for contemporary society. Eerdman listed four reasons that scholars categorize an animal as unclean. He says, "The distinction between clean and unclean animals is arbitrary, cultic, hygienic or symbolic."[30] The hygienic interpretation holds that unclean creatures are unfit to eat because they are carriers of disease ". . . pork can be a source of trichinosis."[31]

Laws are instituted either because of a problem or to prevent one. Again, everything that God created has a particular purpose and should not be altered, in any way to suit humanity's desires. *Funk and Wagnalls* say:

Wild boars were domesticated by Chinese in approximately 2900 B.C. Archaeologists believe that these animals were first domesticated as scavengers and only later to be regarded as food animals.[32]

Henry David Thoreau made a statement that caught my attention, giving me yet a deeper revelation as to why we are to only eat the designated clean animals. He affirms that:

Your body is the temple of God, and His Spirit dwells in you. In the earthy physical temple, do you think they ever brought unclean animals for sacrifice?[33]

Yet men and women of God, who lack the knowledge or clear understanding, are doing it. God only holds us responsible for that which we know and understand. Rev. Dr. Michael Easley, the president of The Moody Bible Institute in

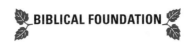

Chicago, made a statement on the radio one morning that resonated with me. He said, "Why we believe what we believe must govern what we do." What one believes is put into practice because the reasoning is trusted and understood. Jordan S. Rubin cites a relevant quote from his book, *The Maker's Diet,* "With impeccable logic, Josephson adds, did anything biologically happen to the swine [since Bible times], or did the digestive tract of man have some sort of miracle transformation?"[34] Rubin goes on to say, "No, the Bible, science and experience have all proven the contrary."[35] Thus, the dialogue this author invites is between Scripture and contemporary cultural understandings.

I am in accord with God's Word being the same yesterday, today and forever (Heb. 13:8), even as God guides His people in the understanding of His mandates as society changes. There need not be a disconnect between the Bible and contemporary times. There simply needs to be revelation regarding that which is hidden in its pages. Gane speaks to that sameness from a contemporary perspective. He says:

> Fortunately, Scripture is not only timely but timeless. Just as God spoke to the original audience, so He still speaks to us through the pages of Scripture. Because we share a common humanity with the people of the Bible, we discover a universal dimension in the problems they faced and the solutions God gave them. The timeless nature of Scripture enables it to speak with power in every time and in every culture.[36]

I understand the New Testament to be a continuation of the Old, or prophecy fulfilled, or that which was concealed to be revealed. The following New Testament scripture will

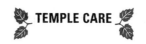

attempt to synthesize the understanding of one's body as presently being God's earthly temple (believers), to be reverenced and cared for as God directs.

1 Corinthians 6:19-20

Or do you not know that your body is a temple of the Holy Spirit within you, which you have from God, and you are not your own? For you were bought with a price; therefore, glorify God in your body.

This particular scripture spoke to my heart for Temple Care because it addresses both spirit and body in the sense of God's dwelling place. Corinth was one of the cities where Paul founded a church. It was located in ancient Greece. It was a commercial city filled with shrines and temples to serve false gods. The goddess of love was the most prominent. It was an important city in Paul's day. However, the culture was corrupt and degraded and full of idolatrous religion. Paul had to address the same kinds of problems a pastor must deal with today, such as carnality and worldliness in the church. Most scholars accept Pauline authorship of 1 Corinthians.

The text speaks to sexual immorality being a sin against one's body (Temple), while other sin is outside of it. The other sins against one's body would include; drugs, suicide, alcohol, smoking, body piercing, gluttony and/or defiling by eating anything that God says is an abomination to His temple. According to David Prior's commentary on the message of 1 Corinthians:

Paul's final plea for purity is based on the cost of redeeming our bodies: you are not your own; you were bought with a price. So glorify God in your body. Before they began to experience the freedom for which Christ had set them free, the Corinthian's were in the most servile bondage. They were slaves to themselves, their self-centered desires, self-indulgence and bodily passions.[37]

In different ways, contemporary culture encourages indulgence in what is not best for the body, and the current secular focus upon morbid obesity (and childhood obesity) demonstrates that. Fast food is everywhere and inexpensive, and has been proven to be unhealthy.

The Corinthians were busy listening to their bodily passions; although, hearing Paul, most weren't listening to the importance of his message from God. Perhaps they weren't "feeling" Paul. Emma J. Justes, author of *Hearing Beyond the Words*, says:

Teenagers today have an interesting way of expressing their understanding of what they have heard: "I feel you.". . . Hearing does not enter into the feeling realm unless it is truly listening.[38]

Paul had a pastor's heart. I could sense his frustration wondering how he could penetrate this near reprobate city. He is listening to God and preaching with every fiber of his being. Leon Morris expresses the complete realm of 1Cor. 6:19-20, when he says:

For the sixth time in this chapter Paul drives home his appeal to what the Corinthians know so well with his argumentative question, Do you not know . . . ? Earlier he referred to the church as a whole as God's temple (3:16), but here body is singular, so that each believer

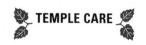

is a temple in which God dwells. The word *naos,* which means the sacred shrine, the sanctuary, the place where deity dwells, not *hieron,* which includes the entire precincts. This gives dignity to the whole of life, such as nothing else could do. Wherever we go we are the bearers of the Holy Ghost, the temples in which God is pleased to dwell. This rules out all such conduct as not appropriate to the temple of God. In application to fornication is obvious, but the principle is of far wider application. Nothing that would be amiss in God's temple in seemly in the child of God.[39]

Amen! A number of pastors today are sharing Paul's sentiment at Corinth exactly with those members of the church whose bodies are there, but their spirits are not. They are hearing messages and leaving the same as before the message (pew warmers). However, when they "feel it," they will be moved by compassion, thereby understanding the sacrifice and love of Jesus that was given to them. They are then moved to change and develop a relationship with Him. In this book, I hope for the readers to "feel" this urgent message of care for the Temple (body) using resources "old" and "new."

I understand the controversy of this message and am prepared to encounter it. As stated in my bio, it is believed that part of the prerequisite to this assignment was clinical pastoral education, which enabled me to disagree agreeably, for such a time as this. I understand there will always be those among us who will not always "feel us," and that's OK! Most importantly, the messenger must bring about delivery of the message, inviting dialogue and openness among different resources and understanding.

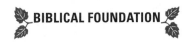

The controversy regarding the food laws has arisen as a result of lack of knowledge and/or understanding of scripture coupled with scientific reasoning. There are many addicted to pork, especially bacon for breakfast or bacon, lettuce and tomato club sandwiches for lunch, and bacon is a staple of "fast food." At issue is not abomination or economics, but the wholeness of the body.

I stopped eating pork in 1972, as stated in my bio, simply for health reasons. Yes, I "heard" of the food laws, however, never with any understanding. I didn't "feel it" until I started preaching "Temple Care" approximately five years ago. I was living it unaware! So, lack of knowledge was part of it for me also, as for all of us who seek a better understanding of our humanness.

African American pastors did not teach the food laws because pork is thought of as an African American food (I will speak to the African American slave diet in the history chapter). So, I began to ask Caucasian pastors, who very much enjoy their summer backyard barbecues, who quickly gave one or the other of the following New Testament scriptures out of context to justify eating pork. Some pastors will quickly preach about deliverance from drugs and alcohol and never mention gluttony. It is the same as drugs; one has to admit the addiction to food before one can be set free (this will be referred to later).

The purpose of using the following four scriptures is for clarification of their true significance. I have selected these particular scriptures because they have often been used in defense of those who say we "no longer live under the law."

By this, I intend to display how scripture can be manipulated to defend one's desires. It is my intention to use the following scriptures in the Temple Care Workbook for new believers' classes and for the "Noble Task," as Dr. Jackie Baston calls it, of reeducating the believers globally. They are as follows: Matthew 15:11-20 (with verse 11 being taken out of context), speaks to the debate over Jewish tradition to wash hands.

In Acts 10:9-34, Peter was very hungry and, therefore, his mind was on food. When he took a nap at the noon hour, and dreamt of the great sheet, he thought God was speaking of food. God spoke to Peter three times saying, "what God has cleansed you must not call common. Peter still thought God was talking about food, when in verse 28, Peter understands that God is speaking to racism, not food.

In 1 Tim. 4:1-5, Paul is warning Timothy of what the false teachers are telling the people so that it could be corrected. It is verse 4 that is taken out of context.

Finally, 1 Corinthians 6:12 is used to say that it's okay to eat anything, just don't over do it.

Morris shed knowledge that allowed a deeper revelation of 1 Cor. 6:12:

> Everything is permissible for me occurs twice here and twice more in 10:23. It looks like a catch-phrase the Corinthians used to justify their conduct . . . But this liberty must be lived out in the spirit of Augustine's maxim, "love, and do what you will." If we love, in the sense in which the New Testament understands love, we need no other guide. The Corinthians, however, were taking Christian liberty to mean, not an unbounded opportunity to show the

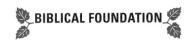

scope of love, but an incredible means of gratifying their own desires.[40]

Augustine was one of the most influential theologians and writers of his time. Having some knowledge of our theological forefathers and foremothers regarding their thinking and integrity helps one to understand why they take a particular stance on a given subject. Augustine was a prisoner to the lust of his flesh before "a work by Cicero converted him to love divine wisdom; but he was repelled by the Bible's apparent barbarity."[41] God chooses one who is less than the best morally so that He, for sure, will get the glory for the transformation as only God can. Nevertheless:

> Augustine raised the self confidence and intellectual lives of African Catholicism under Aurelous Bishop of Carthage 392/2 about 430, councils of bishops again became influential in church life. The councils of Hippo (390) and Carthage, (397) published the first complete canons of the New Testament in the West.[42]

Augustine was Roman Catholic. His written confessions expressed the pain of wrong decisions along life's journey and the peace of developing that true relationship with God that is so liberating. The wonderful thing is that his writing can be instrumental or the catalyst to help someone else out of that same bondage of lust.

Who established the canon?

The councils of Carthage and Hippo did not establish the canon for the church as a whole. The New Catholic Encyclopedia actually affirms the fact that the canon was not officially and authoritatively

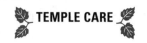

established for the Western Church until the council of Trent in the 16th century and that even such an authority as Pope Gregory the Great rejected the Apocrypha as canonical.[43]

That says to me the 66 books of the Bible are canon.

It may take researching a person or a particular word back to Hebrew and reading it from several Biblical translations for complete understanding of certain scriptural passages. I researched some of the many definitions of the word law in Vine's Bible Dictionary. Two stood out: law of my mind (Rom. 7:23) and exesti (Greek) for lawful; interrogatively to question. Morris continues:

> There is a second reason for caution; I will not be mastered by anything. There is a play on words which Edwards (following Chrisostom) [He was Bishop of Constantinople and a church father of both Roman and Orthodox Christian Traditions], renders all things are in my power, but I shall not be overpowered by anything.[44]

Seeking to follow and understand scripture is a daily walk. Brueggemann agrees that ". . . the Bible is not a drop in activity; it requires a dwelling and a tending over time, a dwelling done in trustful innocence an attending done in critical awareness."[45] With our finite minds, we will never completely understand some of the mandates of our Creator, it is a faith walk. It is my desire that the hearers of Temple Care will understand by faith that whatever is in God's Word is for the good of creation and not harm. Dr. Laura Schlessinger says, "Although we do gain wisdom from the exercise and analysis and discourse of God's commandments, we gain character from our decision to obey in spite of our limited ability to understand."[46] Obedience is much better than sacrifice.

THEOLOGICAL FOUNDATION

My people are destroyed for lack of knowledge. Because you have rejected knowledge, I also will reject you from being priest for me, because you have forgotten the law of your God, I will also forget your children.[1]

God, the Creator, designed and manufactured humans for fellowship. Humanity is:

The highest of God's created beings, who, as created in God's image, have the capacity to be in relationship with God (Gen. 1:26-27) but who, as a result of sin (Gen 3), stand in need of redemption, restoration and salvation found in Jesus Christ.[2]

Health for the human must be defined from a holistic perspective encompassing not only a balance among the spirit, soul and body; it also includes the ethical and social. Somehow, in contemporary society, the physical aspect of that union has been neglected. God said, "Beloved, I pray that all will go well with you and that you may be in good health just as it is well with your soul."[3] Therefore, the best authority to consult regarding holistic care would be the Maker, God.

The Biblical book of Leviticus is that source for God's newly redeemed Hebrew slaves to follow and, I believe, to direct other humans in the universe to adhere to, and be governed by. The laws were for personal and public health along with advice for certain meats from the animal and sea world that would be or not be compatible for human consumption. Meeks gives a crystal clear definition of reasoning behind the food law. He says, "The classification is the result not of empirical medical knowledge but the universal need to classify phenomena by establishing beneficent and destructive categories."[4] Consequently, many people are dying as a result of either not having the knowledge or not understanding it.

The laws were set in motion then and for contemporary times not to return anyone to bondage. I am confident the regulations were established for reasons quite the contrary, to help keep one free from the enslavement of the diseases that may follow as a result of disobedience to God's direction, be it for spiritual, mental or physical well-being. Some of those physical diseases are: diabetes, high blood pressure, heart disease, etc., which are prevalent in America and African Americans who maintain the high-fat diet that was adopted as a result of survival during slavery (see history).

The question was posed to me, "Is Leviticus 'useful' in today's obesity crisis?" Cooti argues that, "A commentary on

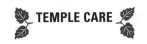

Leviticus must explain convincingly why it is important that this Biblical book should be read today. Unless this question is answered clearly and compellingly, people will not bother to penetrate to its full meaning for today."[5]

The book must not be viewed as simply "food laws," as it is. Gane confirms: "This book of twenty-seven chapters contains more direct speech by God Himself than any other book of the Bible, and is placed at the heart of the Torah or Pentateuch (the five books of Moses), which form the foundation of scripture."[6] God is preparing God's newly redeemed and others to follow this way for relationship, holiness and preparation for His will to be done. R. K. Harrison is fully in accord. He says,

> For the Hebrews to be holy as God is holy requires a close relationship of obedience and faith, and a manifestation in daily life of high moral and spiritual qualities. Characteristic of God's nature as revealed in the law. This same kind of holiness is demanded of every believer in Jesus Christ.[7]

The food laws are simply another external summons by God to live holy in His image and not pollute our bodies with that which is unclean. Today, other pollutants are: drugs, alcohol, cigarettes, gluttony and much more.

Some Christians are full of pride and will not admit they do not know or understand a given Biblical subject. On the other hand, there are those who are humble and open to learn segments of the Bible that have not been previously presented to them. Gane asserts:

. . . Discovering new principles threatens our status quo, especially when they are introduced as "thus saith the Lord." We pay physicians to interfere with our life-styles and counselors to help us adjust. Our Creator gives us prescriptions and counsel free of charge, we tend to resent His meddling and to regard our accountability as a kind of guilt trip. This truth is our responsibility to Him is simultaneously account-ability to ourselves because His instructions are based on cause and effect, like the Surgeon General's recommendation for good diet and exercise and warnings against smoking. Ignorance is blissful as undiagnosed cancer.[8]

In choosing to obey God, the Christian receives an abundant life as a result. Disobedience causes disease and early death.

As a Christian, I was never taught to obey the Biblical diet plan. However, I was impressed from a scientific perspective that the best diet is an abundance of fruits and veggies, with little meat now and then. As stated in the spiritual autobiog-raphy, the choice was made to become a vegetarian because of high-fat content in our diet, and therefore, desiring to eliminate that diet for the purpose of maintaining health.

It dawned on me, while preparing to do my first message on Temple Care, that I had discovered what God desired for me and others to do regarding proper diet through science. With that said, because we are also physical beings, I wondered why the food laws were not part of the founda-tional teaching for the New Believers Class in the Christian church, Bible school or seminary. It appears as though Leviticus is not a part of the canon.

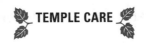

I desired to know the thoughts of other theologians on the subject. So, I e-mailed or called 40 theologians and pastors, some of whom are very renowned. The question posed was: "Have you been taught to live by the Levitical food laws, and do you teach them in your seminary/church?" There were two who responded. I had a sinking feeling this mandate would be challenging.

One of the two who replied was Dr. Jackie Baston, who said, "To reeducate is going to be a noble task!" Those words resonated in my ear as a voice would to one in the wilderness. It is as though Leviticus is a hot potato too many theologians do not want to touch. Just as every knee shall bow and every tongue will confess Jesus is Lord (Rom.14:11), for America to regain the health that is needed, everyone must also become doers of the entire Word, including the food laws.

Some of our theological forefathers and foremothers have shared their impressions regarding the fruits and veggies spoken of in Genesis and specific land and sea animals in Leviticus. Adventists are vegetarian. Ellen G. White, the foundress, gives reasons for discarding flesh. She says:

> Those who eat flesh are but eating grains and vegetables at second hand, for the animals receive from these things the nutrition that produces growth. The life that is in the grains passes into the eater. We receive it by eating the flesh of the animal. How much better to get it directly, by eating the food that God provided for our use![9]

Organic veggies will not have pesticide residue. The meat spoken to above may not contain those nutrients because of hormones and antibiotics or because of what they are fed. One of the reasons why America is constantly gaining weight is very obvious. If the animal is given growth hormones and society eats that animal, guess what? White goes on to say: "Flesh is injurious to health, and whatever affects the body has a corresponding effect on the mind and soul."[10] Daniel speaks to that mental acuity and clear spiritual perception by not defiling his temple with the portion of the king's delicacies (Dan. 1:8-21).

It may appear I am advocating vegetarianism; I am not. I am an advocate of the Word of God, which science has proven to contain the best instruction or guide for the human diet. Because our temple is holy, we must consider how we nourish it. The label says, for best health follow the direction of the designer.

Every home library should have a copy of *The China Study, the Most Comprehensive Study of Nutrition Ever Conducted.* It gives reasons why too much protein (meat) is unhealthy to the human system. Those who chose to eat meat during Biblical times ate very little only on special days or to serve it to a guest in their home. The Campbell's assert that,

> During the past two or three decades, we have acquired substantial evidence that most chronic diseases in America can be partially attributed to bad nutrition. Expert government panels have said it; the surgeon general has said it, and academic scientists have said it. More people die because of the way they eat than from tobacco use, accidents or any other lifestyle or environmental factor. We know that the

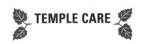

incidence of obesity and diabetes is skyrocketing and that Americans' health is slipping away, and we know what to blame: diet.[11]

Meat, the main culprit, is very heavy on the digestion, is high in fat and processed meat contain nitrites. "Sodium nitrite is a preservative used since the 1920s."[12] According to Campbell's study, "It kills bacteria and adds a happy pink color and desirable taste to hot dogs, bacon and canned meat."[13]

There appears to be an incompatibility with nitrites (a chemical) and the natural human body. Antibiotics and chemotherapy kill bad bacteria and cells. Unfortunately, they also kill the good ones, which explains why a cure in some instances can be just as deadly as the disease. Nitrites have been proven to have a synergistic effect with the body, meaning the two combined may be dangerous. "In 1970, the journal *Nature* reported that the nitrite we consume may be reacting in our bodies to form nitrosamines."[14] Most chemicals are not compatible with the human body and nitrosamines are no exception. The U.S. National Toxicology Program documents that, "No fewer than seventeen nitrosamines are reasonably anticipated to be human carcinogens."[15]

This type of consumer information is usually not a part of the 6 p.m. news. It comes by research because the industry does not want us to know the truth because sales might drop. America's favorite food, the hot dog, could be deadly. Campbell cites from the code of Federal Regulations: Title 9, Animals and Animal Products, "Besides containing additives like nitrites, hot dogs can be made out of ground-up lips, snouts, spleens, tongues, throats and other variety meats."[16]

He went on to share a comment about the hot dog from a presidential candidate. "Ralph Nader had called the hot dogs among America's deadliest missiles."[17] I applaud his statement and therefore concern for humanity. Are nitrite hot dogs a weapon of mass destruction?

Some of our forefathers and foremothers did not have the benefit as we do of scientific study. However, they walked and made decisions by faith and from the similar actions of two or three. Jerome, White and Tertullian were among those theologians who said: "Meat consumption has a great deal to do with lust," and are advocates of vegetarianism and fasting.

Jerome (c. 342-420) was a great scholar who founded monasteries, translated the Bible into Latin, and offended many people with his rigid and extremist views on morality and standards of behavior. Meat for him became a symbol of every kind of self indulgence and lustful desire. Let them eat flesh who serve flesh! Jerome assumes that the human race was originally vegetarian, an assumption that is widely shared in the ancient world. He allowed critics to equate his position with Manichaeism, so that vegetarianism seemed more in tune with distaste for the material world than traditional Christian beliefs about the goodness of creation.[18]

I am in disagreement with Jerome and others who believe that in the beginning, humanity was vegetarian. As stated early on, I have faith that in the beginning humankind was designed to be fruitarian, also eating, nuts

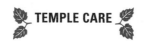

and various grains, using the herbs mostly for medicine that were mostly high in trees because humans are upright. The animals on the other hand walked close to the ground where the vegetables grew naturally for them. It was after the fall when things changed.

Dr. Love, author of *Veggies Suck,* discovered that, "eating red meat actually unleashes testosterone in the male body, which is a major factor behind sexual desires."[19] This appears to be a male only effect. He did not comment on what the findings meant for women. He is certainly encouraging more meat eating. White adds that "flesh food is missed because it is stimulating; it fevers the blood and excites the nerves."[20] Sack made a comment along those lives that spoke to the seriousness of the western diet. He asserts that ". . . the American diet was as scandalous as slavery and drunkenness. With its abundance of meat and grease, it aroused diners' animal passions and destroyed their digestion."[21]

I am a non-denominational Christian and have gleaned knowledge from others who may not believe as I do. All knowledge is precious and turns to wisdom. The Seventh-Day Adventists continue to be leaders in health and prevention.

William Miller, a Baptist minister, predicted that Christ would return in 1843 . . . When the fateful day came and went without the end of history, Miller revised his calculations and predicted a new date the following year. After the second failure, most of Miller's followers fell away. Ellen White, a Millerite and visionary from Maine, organized the faithful remnant under the banner of the Seventh Day Adventist. She argued that meat excited the animal passions. When the animal propensities are increased, she said, the intellectual and moral powers are diseased. The use of the flesh of animals tends to cause a grossness of body, and benumbs the fine sensibilities of the mind.[22]

Meat in moderation appears to be best for those desiring to eat meat, most studies agree. Campbell set out to prove that protein might actually be harmful, and he documents his conclusions:

We now have impressive evidence that low protein intake could markedly decrease enzyme activity and prevent dangerous carcinogen binding to DNA. These were very impressive findings, to be sure. It might even be enough information to "explain" how consuming less protein leads to less cancer.[23]

Christian Americans can be the example for the next generation to follow, either no meat or much less for a healthier society. The churches must serve low-fat potluck meals with an abundance of fruits and veggies.

Tertullian, the father of Latin theology, was born in Carthage, in the province of Africa, around A.D. 150. He was converted to Christianity as a man of about forty. He helped develop the orthodox understanding of the Trinity. He was the first person to use the Latin word *Trinitas* (Trinity). His intellectual brilliance and literary versatility made him one of the most powerful writers of his time and almost as influential as Augustine in the development of Theology in the West.[24]

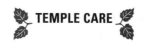
Tertullian wrote a treatise *De Levinio* (on Fasting) . . .
He was critical of gluttony and saw fasting as a way of
drawing closer to God . . ."[25]

Fasting is a topic for another book. However, it is worth
mentioning for the reader as a tool to gain dominion over
one's flesh. I am a firm believer in fasting. Fasting is one of the
best ways to help discipline one's body. That is how I gained
control over my body by fasting every Wednesday on liquids
for years. I grew closer to God and bridled my flesh. Fasting
does not change God: it changes us. Liquid diets (fasts) are
given to patients post surgically in hospitals. "Dr. Howell's
research reveals that whenever the body undergoes fasting,
enzymes normally assigned by the body to digest food are
freed to conduct healing functions, such as dissolving latent
tumors."[26] So, fasting can also aid in the healing process.

Tertullian's quote also mentioned gluttony, a sin seldom
touched from the pulpit.

In fact, many ancient theologians—Ambrose,
Tertullian, John Cuosian and John Chrysostom among
them—equated Adam's original sin, stealing the
forbidden fruit, with gluttony. After all, the very first
rule that God gave humanity was a command of
abstinence, so that controlling one's diet was the
necessary prerequisite to staying in the garden. These
same theologians often took the next step in connect-
ing the sin of fornication with gluttony, if there had
been no gluttony then sexual disorder in excess would
not have entered the world.[27]

The above quote brings to mind Sodom. Overeating is
seen by most in contemporary society as a lack of control, or

an addiction, which appears to be one of the root issues of Sodom. "Look, this was the iniquity of your sister Sodom: She and her daughter had pride, fullness of food and abundance of idleness; neither did she strengthen the hand of the poor and needy."[28] That is clearly saying we must become doers of the Word and not just hearers only, in every way. "Truth that is not lived, that is not imparted, loses its life-giving power, its healing virtue."[29] It appears the focus was on satisfying the pleasures of the body where seeds were planted instead of towards spiritual growth.

Our theological forefathers and foremothers have paved the way historically for us to continue, generation after generation, to have a better cognitive understanding of the Biblical, spiritual laws. That perception allows one to see (feel) the scarlet thread (the continued, unbroken connection) between then and now (them and us). Historian David Hackett Fischer adds to that. "History can be useful as history in several substantial ways. It can serve to clarify contexts in which contemporary problems exist."[30] Understanding the intended diet plan from Biblical history will help one to better understand the obesity epidemic that is bordering on pandemic, which is existing especially in America today.

HISTORICAL FOUNDATION

Science has proven direction pertaining to health in every area of human existence is hidden in the ancient Biblical scriptures. Reginald Cherry, a Christian medical doctor, substantiates through his personal research that "Woven into ancient Hebrew, Aramaic and Greek manuscripts are clues to health and healing only recently validated by scientific medical research."[1] When Cherry was a science major training to become a medical doctor, he: ". . . was astonished by the ways dietary and nutritional laws given in the ancient Biblical texts revealed truths that scientists were only beginning to uncover in this century."[2] A question comes to mind about other not as important manuals, such as those for computers, copiers, scanners, games, toys and again, especially one's automobile, that are never questioned or attempted to be proven. They are simply followed by faith because no one knows a product better than its creator. The dietary plans were set in place before man/woman was created. However, the manuals were given later by inspiration (see Biblical foundation). Proper Temple Care is done according to the Creator's specifications in His Word. The Relationship of Temple Care to Improved Health Status for Individuals Afflicted with Obesity is certainly what has been addressed. This historical study will look to the Biblical food history, understanding that humans are exclusively historical beings. The purpose of this search is to find "That which is accepted as being historically true because it is based on verifiable facts and accounts."[3] Along with this journey of historicity, the following reports will chronicle information that will assist one with the grounding and therefore provide a support base for the understanding of this work. I will touch on the following questions as food for thought. A Biblical history of food will be the first stop. Moving on, the question of when the Christians separated from the Jews will be answered. I say separate and not divorce because the Pentateuch remained a part of foundational Christian teaching although; Leviticus appears not to be a part of the canon. What did Jesus eat is a question that will be addressed, along with the importance of dining together. Feasting, as known in Biblical history, has continued in the church today, only the contents are much more deadly. The African American slave diet will be addressed along with its significance to contemporary African American health. This journey will end with an answer to the question, "What can the consumer do today to 'stop' the food manufacturers from including additives and other harmful chemicals to our food source that will lessen obesity and increase health?"

What comes to mind historically first about food is how God rained manna [Exodus 16] and quail from heaven to feed the Israelites in the wilderness, which is understood as a

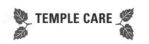

miracle. *The Frugal Gourmet,* who was a chaplain and Methodist pastor calls manna, "grain from heaven."[4] Manna fell from the heavens and had to be collected daily as directed by God. "The word for 'what is it?' in Hebrew is *manna.*"[5] Smith expands that definition another step: "What is it comes from the Hebrew phrase, *"man-hu."*[6] Colbert went on to explain the constituents of manna, which certainly helps with understanding the importance of bread then and now. He says:

> Manna appeared to them to be like small, round coriander seeds, as fine as frost. It was the color of baellium—a pearlized white color. The people could cook it like grain-grind it on millstones or beat it in a mortar, and then cook it in pans or make cakes from it. It had the taste of "pastry prepared with oil" or "wafers" made with honey (Num. 14:8; Ex. 16:31).[7]

The Israelites knew if they were not obedient to the collection process, "any manna left on the ground melted in the heat of the desert sun."[8] Smith shares yet another representation of manna. He found that it:

> . . . Was also a symbol for the fact that no matter what kind of jam we get ourselves into, the Holy One will be there ahead of us, along with manna from Heaven that we probably don't deserve. Bread and grain are also used to teach us about our responsibility to our fellow men and women. Do not harvest the whole of the field, but leave the corners for the wandering hungry that will come by (Deut. 24:19). So why is the farmer responsible for the hungry? Because he has grain, and must not keep it all for himself? Bread

teaches us that we must feed each other or some of us will die.[9]

During Biblical times, the weight was controlled by most of society because the food was regulated. The diet was simple and consistent from a basic food plan. The foods we get today from that basic food plan are:

Cereal grains are among man's oldest foods, and the biblical peoples, grain of life. The worst revenge an enemy could wreak was to sow weeds among the wheat and thus strangle the season's food supply.[10]

Staple foods are survival foods and/or basic foods to build on or start from. The Israelites survived on the grain; therefore, it had to be packed with the necessary nutrients to sustain health and therefore life, as others have realized.

Every day one ate pretty much the same thing. Bread, salt [natural], milk and honey, olive oil, and of course wine. During a very good week you might have some dried fish or olives. Meat was eaten only on High Holy Days. The diet was bread, oil and wine three times a day. Perhaps some cheese would show up now and then but we must remember that such things were very scarce unless you were wealthy and of the ruling class.[11]

Regarding wine, when Paul said to Timothy, "No longer drink only water, but use a little wine for your stomach's sake and your infirmities" (1Tim. 5:23), he could have been saying that wine is medicine. Doesn't infirmity mean "any medical condition that causes a lack of strength or vitality?"[12] Many researchers have discovered the health properties in red

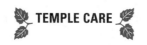

wine, be it with alcohol or non-alcoholic. Dr. Reginald Cherry discovered red wine contains resveratral.

> Researchers at the University of Illinois have found that resveratral inhibits cancer by helping to prevent DNA damage to cells, keeping cells from transforming into cancer, and thus preventing the growth and spread of cancer. Resveratral has been shown to lower cholesterol in recent Cornell University students.[13]

It is also said to be packed with antioxidants. Wine produced from organic grapes would certainly be the best.

One of the Biblical grains that serves as a staple today is corn. Many of our cereals are made from these same grains, the corn flake.

> ... The term corn in the English spoken at the time [*Beaucal*] referred to any and all grains; just as our term grain covers all sorts of cereals...maize was given the name corn, or grain, by the English settlers. So, while corn is mentioned in the King James Version of the Bible, it was not corn as we know it but simply grain.[14]

Ellen White, the foundress of the Seventh-Day Adventist vision, encompassed the entire health of a human being. Therefore, she was concerned about one's diet. Health reform was a part of her vision that went beyond diet. Members of her organization shared that vision with that same passion for care.

> In 1876 John Harvey Kellogg, a member of the church, became director of the institute, later known as the Battle Creek Sanitarium—the san for short.[15]

It appears there was a noticed correlation by Dr. Kellogg between disease and certain foods consumed before and during her reign that both she and Dr. Kellogg were concerned about. "In 1895 the doctor and his brother, W. K., invented the corn flake, a grain meant to replace meat on the breakfast table."[16] Too much meat consumption was apparently creating related diseases as it is today on a grand scale.

The Israelites murmured because they missed the meat they ate in Egypt. Therefore, God showered quail from heaven. They had meat and bread. God gave them a diet plan that would be best for them, including the best meat to eat, because they simply didn't know (see Bible). Lise Stern, in her book *How to Keep Kosher*, says: "No forbidden meat, fowl or seafood (the list includes pork, birds of prey and shellfish."[17] Stern mentioned a bit of history in her book that may shed another ray of light of understanding on the food law subject. She mentioned the importance of a historical and important Rabbi called Rambam:

> Rambam, the name of honor given to Rabbi Mashe ben Maimon, also called Maimonide, was a twelfth century scholar and physician who lived in Cairo. Rambam is most known for his fourteen-volume *mishneh* Torah. *Mishneh Torah* can mean "repetition of the Torah"; his work incorporates both the written and oral Torah.[18]

It appears the laws were accepted by faith. She goes on to say:

> . . . Rambam himself offered a few reasons for the dietary *mitzvoth;* that God, in making the laws, was considering both our moral and physical beings. In

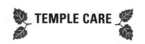

his *Guide to the Perplexed,* Rambam wrote that *Kashrut* [keeping it kosher] trains us to master our appetites; to accustom us to restrain our desires; and avoid considering the pleasure of eating and drinking as the goal of man's existence.[19]

In agreement with most scholars, the food laws are to strengthen and protect us from impurities. Wayne Daniel Bernard adds:

Many who consider themselves good Jews do not follow *Kashrut* or do so in rudimentary form-not eating pork, perhaps, or leaving cheese off the hamburger. Only the most extreme orthodox would assert that such people are not truly Jews.[20]

That same mandate is for the Christian. After all, we are Judeo-Christians. Jesus is a Jew.

Muslims are also very serious about adhering to their dietary laws, especially regarding swine and what basically appears to be the same reasoning as the Bible. The Qur'an, the Muslims holy book, says this regarding meat that should not be eaten:

God has only forbidden you *carrion* [rotting animal flesh of a dead animal], and blood and flesh of swine [swine, consumes carrion], and that over which other than God has been invoked. But there is no transgression or blame on those who are compelled by necessity, without wanting or going too far. For God is most forgiving and most merciful.[21]

When God gave the law, it was for the universe, which includes all of human kind. "Ancient Egyptians, unlike their modern Muslim descendents, had a taste for pork, according to a mummy autopsy."[22] These findings are mentioned simply to reiterate the dangers of pork consumption can be traced in history. "A pathologist from Italy's Pisa University, and a colleague report the discovery of the oldest known case of cysticercosis—a pig-related-disease in a mummy from the late phatemiac period (II-I Century B.C.)."[23]

If Christianity was birthed out of Judaism, then why do Christians not observe the food laws? The first church family split did not occur between the Catholics and Lutherans. It was the separation of Christians and Jews. I say separate and not divorce because Christians adhere to other areas of the Judeo-Christian Word, perhaps that which is most comfortable. So that says to me that, be it conscious or subconscious, we remain spiritual family because of Jesus, who is a Jew. Does the separation explain why Leviticus appears not to be a part of the canon? Wayne Daniel Berard gives meaning to those important questions from history in his book, *When Christians Were Jews.* "For in 70, the overwhelming majority of those who believed in Jesus were Jews who saw themselves as such."[24] That was part of the concern that the Jews were going to take over using the name of Jesus, and were therefore, forbidden to use that name (Acts 4:16-18).

> At the time of the creation of Mark there was no such thing as Christianity as we conceive of it today. There were Jews who believed that Jesus was the Messiah...Hence, the world to which Mark's Gospel is addressed is one in which Christians were Jews or largely of Jewish consciousness . . . Jews that believed in Jesus regularly worshipped in the Temple and

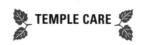

followed the mosaic practice of sacrifice. They did not see themselves as a separate people or religion for which the destruction of the Temple had no meaning. In fact, as witnessed by Mark, the "Jesus Jews" had an answer they wished to propose to question of why God had permitted this catastrophe to happen. It was over this very question and competing answers which emerged between 70 and 90 C.E. that the family split in Judaism occurred.[25]

The answer to why Christians do not observe the Levitical laws is so simple, yet so profound. As Christians, we must remember that we are spiritual Jews. Berard documents,

> Christians for two millennia have endeavored to imitate Christ-in all but his inclusive Judaism. Nowhere in the Gospel does Jesus ever "enforce" any of His teachings, not the most central truth, the most beneficial practice. He never expels any of his error-prone disciples, not even his own betrayer. Rather in the tradition of his Jewish faith, Jesus teaches, just teaches, and believes that if the teaching, is truly the Word of God it will not need enforcement; it will grow like the parable's seed in the night, one knows not how. In Judaism, one does not need to enforce the faith as taught; one's faith is in the teachings.[26]

The question is, as Judeo-Christians, do we need to ask forgiveness for not adhering to part of the Word unaware? It is my desire to shed light through *Temple Care Workbook* for new believers to understand Leviticus is also a part of the Bible to adhere to. Through that adherence, the next generation of Christians and those who follow by example will be much healthier.

Jesus was our example in every way when He walked the earth fully man and fully God. He was not only our model for faith and integrity, but how He cared for Himself physically was also a representation for us to emulate. What did Jesus eat?

> In the ancient near East, two meals were normally eaten during the day. The first was the noonday meal, usually consumed by laborers in the field and consisting of such items as small cakes or flat loaves, figs or olives and possibly curds of goat milk. Breakfast was considered unnecessary, and Biblical references to any such forms of early meals are few (Kgs. 19:5; John 21:12). Among the Hebrews, the evening meal was the most important occasion of the day. The meal was eaten together by the entire family. There was no separate dining room in the average house and during the Patriarchal period, meals were consumed while sitting in Egyptian fashion in a reclining position became popular, and continued through the Roman period.[27]

Fish was also part of Jesus' diet and culture, especially from the miracle of feeding over five thousand from two fish (Matt. 14:14-20). Naomi Goodman documents in *The Good Book Cook Book* that:

> The fish predated the cross as the first symbol of the early Christian church. The Greek word for fish, *icthus,* was read as an acrostic for Jesus Christ, Son of God, and Savior. Because of this association and many references to fish in the New Testament, it was a popular food with Christians.[28]

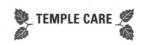

The best was served to guests, therefore, Jesus, as a guest no doubt was served beef or lamb from time to time. Hands were used for utensils. Like churches today, celebrations centered around food in Biblical times.

References to food and related themes appear in every book of the Bible starting with Genesis and ending in Revelation 22. Indeed, some of the best stories are those dealing with food and food getting. O.T. examples: Eve's temptation of Adam, Joseph saving the people of Egypt and his own family from famine; Boaz' field, Elisha who kept the widow's oil flowing, the young Hebrew boys who would not eat the King's unclean food.[29]

I am also reminded of the feast for the return of the prodigal son. Those same feasts have continued in the churches today: ordinations, weddings, graduations, etc. Sometimes, there is simply a once-a-month community "potluck" feast. "Food consumed communally, as understood in Bible times, made you a member of that same family or tribe."[30] Our feasts today consist of the meals that are not as healthy as they were in Bible times. Food basically has the same meaning for the various cultures. The meals are just different. Smith adds, "Food functioned in the Bible as a means of communication, and the table became the symbol of intimacy. Indeed, eating with someone at the table was considered more intimate than sexual involvement."[31]

The culture of Pompeii 2000 years ago was discovered by archaeologists in the ruins after the eruption of Mt. Vesuvius in 79 A.D. What they ate was found in the sewage system, which was also used for a garbage deposit, in which were found grape seeds, apple pits and fig seeds. They also found loaves of bread intact in ovens.

> Pompeii's busiest restaurant was buried with the rest of the prosperous city when Mount Vesuvius erupted in A.D. 79. The eruption killed thousands of people, but a 20-foot-deep (6 meter-deep) cocoon of volcanic ash kept the city almost intact, providing precious information on domestic life in the ancient world.[32]

The article went on to confirm that "cereals and beans were staples of the Roman diet, together with fish, cheese and limited quantities of eggs and meat."[33]

That passion today has moved to addiction for some. We must also reach out to our church family members and again by example encourage low-fat potluck meals and more fruits and vegetables, along with exercise. Pastors must address gluttony for the sin that it is and what it is doing universally. Relationships are also built at church potluck dinners. Some churches are known for the lavish, tasty, high-fat meals. I spoke at one such church recently and was asked not to mention food. My spirit sank. Although I did not plan to mention anything about food, it is comparable to having members that you know are living together outside of marriage. After all now, we don't want to offend. Maybe it's one of the good tithing trustees and you're asked not to mention fornication, what's the difference? Sin is sin according to God's Word. Gluttony is sin.

Obesity stats are climbing yearly. I have a passion to leave a legacy that will reverse those stats for generations to come. For example,

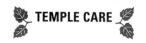

In 1901, the United States was classified as the healthiest nation in the world among one hundred nations. By 1920, we had dropped to second place. By 1950, we were in third place. By 1970, were in forty-first place. And by 1981, we had dropped all the way to ninety-fifth place.[34]

What happened so fast? Why is it that people from outside of America are slim and trim until they move to America? It appears that, as the importance of family and eating together declined, fast foods increased. Normal servings are not enough; everything has a biggie size, and has been cooked in trans-fat, which is not compatible for healthy arteries (as of this printing, a law requires that trans-fat not be used in any fast food restaurants).

Health care cost is also on the rise and hurts everyone financially. According to Eric Neuberger, executive director for the Indiana Governors council for Physical Fitness and Sports says: "Indiana has among the highest health care cost in the nation."[35] Indiana has moved from the 3rd most obese state down to the 11th, according to the Center for Disease Control (CDC). There is no one single area to blame for this obesity epidemic; however:

> Most scientists blame the epidemic of serious diseases on processed foods. These adverse health conditions include this top fifteen list: obesity, heart disease, cancer, diabetes, hypertension, high cholesterol, attention deficit disorder, gastro esophageal reflux, gallbladder disease, diverticulosis, arthritis, chronic fatigue syndrome, fibromyalgia, and addictions.[36]

The focus of this work is obesity in America, which is the cause for most of the health issues named above. However, I have a particular concern about the African-American diet, which is high in fat. Although in the minority, they suffer as a whole a high percent of the disease processes named above because of diet. Some of the staggering statistics include:

78% of African American females, 60% of African American males, 74% Hispanic American females, and 72% of Hispanic males are overweight or obese (Center for Disease Control). 1 out of 4 adults in the U.S. are obese. 18-20% of children in U.S. are obese. About 40% of obese children and about 80% of obese adolescents become obese adults.[37]

Statistics have kept us informed that America is getting more and more obese. African American females are at the top of that list. Just as one's personality, "a person's food preferences are actually formed during the first four to five years of life."[38] Children either were not introduced to it when young or someone else disliked that particular food. History is part of one's culture and can certainly have an adverse or positive effect.

Lee H. Butler Jr., in his book, *Loving Home,* asserts that:

The activities of each generation affect the lives of the generations that follow. Everyone has been influenced by the lives of those who have walked ahead of us. Our present attitudes have been shaped by those who first lived the African-American experience. Parents influence children, and older siblings influence younger siblings. Acts of protest and violence affect those directly involved as well as those who were not

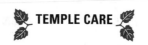

present. What we do today will influence the lives of those who will be responsible tomorrow.[39]

This quote says to me the history of the family is of great importance for survival. What is passed on generation after generation should aid in a people's strengthening, not in their demise. The African American diet and inactivity is causing some of the above-named diseases, such as diabetes, high blood pressure, high cholesterol, heart disease and cancer because of the high animal fat content in the diet.

Knowing one's history in a given area, especially if it has been a detriment or is found to be one, should be reason not to repeat it. Not having knowledge of one's personal, cultural and historical background as it relates to a given area, in this illustration which is food, would become a future detriment. Having learned of a prejudicial situation that has become ingrained as part of one's culture, to continue that self infliction is akin to suicide. Acting on that insight to change one's diet is wisdom.

The African American diet during slavery was discarded pork and vegetable parts. That diet from being enslaved has become what I call a "generational curse." African Americans are survivors as a people, therefore, are pliable and can adjust to the situation by the grace of God, as Paul says:

> I know how to be abased, and I know how to abound. Everywhere in all things I have learned both to be full and be hungry, both to abound and suffer need I can do all things through Christ who strengthens me (Phil. 4:12-13).

Actually, the southern white slave owners did not realize all of swine was garbage when they gave the slaves hocks, feet, ears, chitlins, etc., which is a culprit of contemporary obesity and the above-named diseases. African Americans added soul and a particular flavor to the above-named foods that made it not only palatable, but pleasing. This, over the years, has become "soul food."

The "soul" ingredient of the meal certainly comes from the cook. We are spirit, soul and body. One's soul is one's mental and emotional side that determines and does the will of God, when it has been renewed by God's Word. Although the slaves were illiterate and not allowed to learn to read, God was certainly in their hearts and kept them going because He is the God of the oppressed (Ps. 103:6). The love of God and the love of family motivated the cooks during slavery to pray and sing various hymns as they lovingly added the various spices they were impressed to add. If the slaves were able to read the Levitical food laws regarding pork, they would not have been able to comply because that was what they survived on. And yes, God would have forgiven them if they had known.

The slaves were very active in the fields doing whatever labor they were assigned from sunup to sundown. That hard labor is what kept some of the same above named diseases from inflicting the slaves. Again, food was one of the few pleasures when they gathered together. Soul food has been around for generations. However, "soul food was given to the African American style of cooking in the sixties when the word soul became associated with most things African

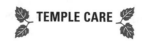

American."[40] That says to me a survival food has been accepted as culture.

In the 60's era, being black and proud removed the stigma of inferiority while attempting to move into the ranks of equality. When someone talks about African American food, they may not say African American food; however, when they say soul food, that is what is meant.

> The roots of soul food can be traced back to Africa. African slave leaders brought food over to America from Africa along with the slaves. It is thought that some slaves brought seeds of native crops along with them to America, hiding the seeds in their ears and hair. Some of these foods became part of America's food crops and food. Using discarded meat from the plantations like pig's feet, ham hocks, chitterlings (pig small intestines) pig ears, hog jowls, tripe and skin, cooks added onion, garlic, thyme and bay leaf to enhance the flavor. The slaves were also given discarded tops of vegetables like the tops of beets and dandelions. These items can be found in many soul food dishes today.[41]

That is called making the best of what one has (making-do). "Dick Gregory condemned the "slave" diet as an unclean and/or unhealthful practice of racial genocide."[42] Actually, in analyzing the diet today according to scientists, it was not totally destructive. As mentioned, field exercise was one reason. The soil contained many more pure nutrients then; therefore, their vegetable garden, although they received what was discarded, was full of nutrients. Onions are said to fight cancer, garlic is good for high blood pressure and cholesterol, thyme has antiviral properties and the bay leaves helped to maintain an alkaline PH. So, the nutrients helped balance the negative mainly because the exercise maintained good circulation: therefore, a stronger immune system was able to continue to fight.

The Bible specifically instructs us not to eat fat or blood (Lev. 3:17). Animal fat is saturated and dangerous to humanity. Pork has fat throughout the meat. Dr. Reginald Cherry suggests for men that "Avoiding foods with saturated [animal fat] fats also provides protection against prostate cancer."[43] For women, the fat has growth hormones that have been linked to breast cancer. God was on to something!

William C. Whit gives another definition of culture that is worth mentioning:

> Culture originates as an attempt to come to terms with an environment's physical and social aspects. As a system of human interactions, however, culture does more than reflect adaptation. Rather, it is an adaptive response. That term denotes both an active, creative human involvement and a dialectical interplay between human actor and environment.[44]

This helps explain how the African American diet was adopted and passed on generation after generation as culture. More questions need to be asked about the diet in Africa before slavery took place. The only thing that can be worse than the degradation of "giving" a human one's garbage to eat is to "sell" it to them. After the Emancipation Proclamation, so-called freedom, with no education or ability to get jobs, African-Americans were poor. After the slaves were set free from bondage, the pork meat parts that were once discarded, nevertheless free, now had to be purchased. Again, the focus was on survival. Therefore, they had to resort to other "abominable" foods they gathered by fishing or hunting, such as catfish and rabbit. The white-owned stores in the north that were located in the African American neighborhoods sold the inferior meat (not fresh, repackaged after three days in the white store and moved to the African American store to sell), and other food products. The inferior cuts along with chitterlings (chitlins) were sold only in African American stores at one time. For fresh meat and produce, the African American had to travel across town to the white supermarkets (which I lived through as a child and adult).

African Americans are no longer enslaved physically. However, some are still bound subconsciously many generations later by the same diet that is not only causing health demise, but goes against the directions of God. Akbar NA'IM expresses this sentiment well in his book, *Breaking The Chains of Psychological Slavery.* He says,

> The intensity and brutality of the slave-making experience traumatized our social and human development. Though many writers have spoken of slavery, few scholars have addressed the continuity of the behaviors established in slavery as a continuing aspect of African-American psychology.[45]

Again, that also says to me a renewing of one's mind is vital. The participants in the Temple Care Workshop did not find that adjustment difficult at all. In fact, they welcomed it for health benefits. Rabbi Plotkin says, "If you want to do something, it's never hard. If you don't, it's overwhelming."[46] By the grace of God, one can comply with God's Word.

Obesity is costly; however, eating healthy is also costly. Obesity's cost could be one's life as a result of one of the named diseases and health care expenses. Eating organic costs more financially; however, in the long run it pays off in health benefits. Since church is home away from home, if the fat is cut at home for health, it should be encouraged to be cut at church. Since Christians are the majority of people in America, we can then make the obesity stats healthier.

What can individuals do with the information received? As consumers, how can we encourage manufacturers to return to raising animals in a healthy manner?

People have tried many different programs but to no avail. Dr. Ben Lerner spoke to that issue in his book, *Body by God.* He says, "The reason most health books and positive mental attitude programs fail to create any long-term success is that the information is only man's and little is God's."[47] The only true success in proper diet and any other areas of life comes from doing it God's way, setting the example for generations to come. Continuing with that same sentiment, Ellen White affirms that "truth that is not lived, that is not imparted, loses its life-giving power, its healing virtue."[48]

Scientists say the best diet for humanity is plenty of fruits and veggies and a little meat two or three times a month as a side dish. The Creator (God) says eat plenty of fruits and veggies and the little meat, if you choose to eat it, should be selected from the clean list, as a side dish or two or three times

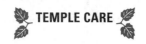

a month. One could simply choose as Daniel to be vegetarian. They are all healthy choices when kept in moderation.

We must come together as consumers to stop meat packers and farmers from putting deadly additives in our food. "In 1991, the Centers for Disease Control (CDC) released a startling statistic-approximately half of the fifteen million pounds of antibiotics produced annually in America are used to treat livestock and poultry."[49] Is that because they are inhumanely crowded together and may catch each other's diseases? If consumers band together and have a mass exodus from purchasing poison meat, they will stop poisoning it. That happened with success with the "alar" case. Alar was reported on *60 Minutes:* "The most potent carcinogen in the food supply."[50] Alar was sprayed on apples as a growth regulator.

> The public reaction was swift. One woman called the state police to chase down a school bus to confiscate her child's apple. School systems across the country in New York, Los Angeles, Atlanta and Chicago, among others, stopped serving apples and apple products. According to John Rice, former chairman of the U.S. Apple Association, the apple industry took an economic walloping, losing $250 million. Finally, in response to the public outcry, the production and use of alar came to a halt in June 1989.[51]

America came together as a team then, so that proves we can do it again.

6

THEORETICAL
FOUNDATION

I can do all things through Christ who strengthens me!

Phil. 4:13

Habit is habit and not to be flung out of the window by any man [woman], but coaxed downstairs a step at a time.

Mark Twain

If you don't do what is best for your body you're the one who comes up with the short end.

Julius Erving

Motivation is the primary component needed to accomplish and master a lifestyle diet change. Victory is inclusive with the self-confidence built mainly on Biblical principles. I am not talking about the spirit of energy that comes with making New Year's resolutions that fizzle before or by spring. Neither am I speaking of a quick fix to get into an outfit for a special occasion, such as class reunion, birthday, anniversary, New Year's Eve, weddings and such. Then, after the event, the weight returns with a large bonus.

Diets are always short term. A lifestyle change endures for the long haul. It becomes automatic because of a renewed mind. The eating habits are aimed toward health and healing, not feeling. The standard prescribed orders were written in the Bible. Theory has described the reasoning behind the Creator's writing the mandate is to benefit humanity and not harm it, as not adhering to it has caused His Creation.

The Biblical, Theological and Historical foundations spoke to the theory of America bordering upon a pandemic of obesity and offered solutions both Biblical and scientific regarding diet reform. When one knows better, one usually does better in God's timing. We are responsible for that which we know and have a basic understanding of. That discernment adds to one's motivational process.

Science is "the study of the physical world and its manifestations, especially by using systemic observation and experiment."[1] Scientists have proven the origin of humanity through DNA studies that the Bible is what it says it is, and archaeologists have discovered the diet of humanity during Bible times 2000 years ago. Today, scientific theory and the American Cancer Society are amazingly on one accord regarding that same standard Biblical food prescription for health and healing. That diet includes plenty of fresh, raw fruits and veggies with a little meat as a side dish, if one desires. Pork is deemed too fat scientifically and unclean Biblically. One of the Biblical mandates is not to eat animal fat. We can observe around us what causes the obesity America is faced with. Olive oil is the oil used in Biblical times and scientifically suggested to use today. It fights bad cholesterol. God was on to something!

Our theological forefathers and foremothers have assisted with the understanding of the use of Biblical theory from his/her expertise. God desires for us to be doers of the Word and not hearers only. They have helped us put theory to use in a contemporary setting, with each one building on the formers knowledge to our gain. Medical doctors and other writers have certainly helped clarify the best diet for humanity.

History has been proven to repeat itself, whether negative or positive. The positive should continue to get stronger, generation after generation. The negative can only get worse and must not only be stopped; nonetheless the seed of its inception must be uprooted. An example is the high fat pork diet from slavery in the history of the African American. Theory has shown whatever has been programmed into one's mind from one's culture from birth to five not only forms one's personality, but also the eating habits. Therefore, one's mind must be reprogrammed for healthy eating habits. James Cone cites a quote from Werner Starks that clarifies that statement. Werner Starks says, "We see through the broad and deep acres of history through a mental grid . . . through a system of values which is established in our minds before we look out on to it—and it is this grid which decides . . . what will fall into our field of perception."[2] That grid is analogous to a computer program that simply needs to be reprogrammed with healthy information. Until that change occurs, one will automatically continue the same historical habits.

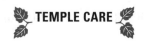

It is my desire that something was said biblically, theologically or historically in theory that will trigger the reader's enthusiasm and aid in a healthy lifestyle change and assist with the Bible making more sense. Hopefully, this foundation will be the driving force, the seeds of knowledge, reasoning and support that will build the self-confidence for victory along with the Temple Care Workshop.

As a motivational tool I am closing this chapter with the personal testimonies of Dr. Karen Edwards and Mrs. Brenda Harvey who were both presenters for the workshop.

Karen Edwards is a Doctor of Naturopathy/Herbologist. Her ministry gradually came into existence as a result of seeking treatment for herself. As a child/preteen, she was diagnosed with type I diabetes. She started taking shots early in life. During those years, she instinctively began to eat differently than the Doctors informed. She was told to eat "diabetic" foods and count food exchanges. She says, with diabetes, life revolves around your food intake, shots and the ups and downs of the disease.

She began looking at the food labels and realized-there is really not food in there! It is all chemicals, dyes and synthetic material. She started eating "real" food-the whole food-the whole food that is God-given and grown from the earth: vegetables, fruits, seeds, nuts, beans and legumes. The packaged diabetic foods were all full of aspartame and synthetic sweeteners, which she now understands to be one of the biggest disease inducers in our country. But as a young girl, she had no clue why she was choosing that way of eating. She said meat was removed from her diet, not intentionally, but intuitively. She started loving nuts and seeds, where she received much of her protein. According to her junk food friends, she ate some pretty strange foods that were not on the Standard American Diet (SAD) of chemically laden packed foods.

Her father was a Christian and was always there for her. As a child, he would pray for her sore throats, stomach aches and ailments and tell them "just believe that you are healed, and God will take care of it." He joked about some of the food she concocted.

Throughout the early adult years, she had complications with pregnancies, a very early hysterectomy and numerous surgeries attributed to diabetes. Miraculously, she has two wonderful children. The surgery followed immediately after her youngest son was born. The diabetes became more rigid and she developed the usual eye, heart and kidney problems many diabetics come to know over time. The ritual of living life around her shots was growing old. She was imagining life as a non-diabetic. She was hospitalized three times a year minimum, for many years.

Medical doctors told her to get her life in order and make necessary arrangements for her children. She was told her disease was so progressive, she would not live to see 30 (she was then 25). The way it was going, she said that appeared to be the case. She weighed 90 pounds tops. She was adamant about eating right, but many times thought if she were going to die soon anyway, why not self destruct now (another typical attitude of diabetics)? She would sneak a whole pie into the bathroom and eat it, or a Snickers bar. She realized

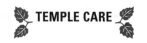

this was not the answer. Good diet ended up winning out, because that is what she really believed in. She said God gave her the right choices to go on. She had to stay true to her intuition and not her "taste buds." Food is fuel. The higher quality the food with live enzymes and minerals, the more life giving fuel you get in return.

In 1989, she lived in California, her dad grew ill and her emotions were high. This increased the severity of the diabetes. In June 1990, he passed away. Through her hysteria and pain, she became numb. She could not eat or make arrangements to go home. Her colleagues put together her flight and reminded her of the importance of eating and taking her shots because of her disease (they all knew the repercussions when she missed a meal or a shot).

In that instant, God graced her with one of the greatest gifts. He gave her the faith to KNOW His Word still stands the SAME today as it always had. She remembered the times sitting on her father's lap, and he loved her so much to ask God to remove her sore throats or whatever it was. She had the faith a child has, to believe God took it away and she went on about her business playing and never looked back. She said, unbeknownst to her friends and family, she asked that morning for God to remove her diabetes and accepted that by His stripes it was ALREADY taken away (1 Peter 2:24). She just had to accept it. She had faith that was beyond what she has ever known since. She threw away her insulin [she is not advocating anyone do this], syringes and heart medicine. From that moment, she has never had another medicine for those diseases. She is in medical books as a Miraculous Healing, because science cannot explain it at all.

Throughout the years, she has continued to practice a "Whole Health" diet and lifestyle. She realizes you don't have to have a disease to eat the foods God designed to keep our bodies healthy. She said was God's original plan all along. She began to study nutrition and herbs and now is a doctor of naturopathy and has a degree as a herbologist, and degrees in iridology and sclerology.

Dr. Karen went on to explain to the group the basic tenet of naturopathy is that human life is governed by the same self-repairing forces that care for all living things. The methods are natural and utilize readily available God-given resources such as pure food, water, liquid and oxygen. These improvements in daily lifestyle support the "whole" body in healing from within using nontoxic therapies. She said it is the naturopath's job to sort out the pure and help us eliminate the chemicals, xenotoxins, excretoxins and life's negative agents that cause so much stress, disease and depression abundant in our society.

She stressed it is not a one size fits all. It is treated as any other medical specialty. She has assisted many physicians with situations that were difficult, with very positive results. She can be reached at herbdoc@comcast.net.

Any program of this magnitude must have a heartfelt counselor, one who has suffered the pain of obesity and has the victory. Brenda Harvey is a Biblical counselor and a member of the American Association of Christian Counselors. Personal journeys out of food addictions can be a strength for others. Mrs. Harvey shared some of her counseling stories at

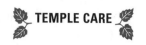

the workshop to encourage others. Neil Anderson is quoted from his book Bondage Breaker:

> The basis for temptation is legitimate human needs. We will either look to the world, the flesh and the devil to have our needs met, or we will look to Christ who promises to meet our needs (Phil 4:19). The essence of temptation is the invitation to live independently of God.[3]

She also agrees it began in the garden. The temptation was to live independently of God by eating a piece of fruit. The temptation is there to meet our own needs without looking to the Creator to meet our needs. The temptation to say "I can do this myself, I don't need God." The temptation is also there to be self sufficient rather than Christ-sufficient, the temptation to gratify our flesh, our pride, immediately rather than waiting on God. It began in the garden and it began for Brenda at the age of 5.

That was when her whole world turned upside down and she had legitimate, unmet needs. The adults in her life became emotionally and physically unavailable. Her father was absent and her mother became an emotional cripple. The adults (grandparents and neighbors) who were in her life believed if she had food in the house, they were taking care of her. People said to Brenda, "Here honey, have something to eat, it will be okay," and it wasn't. She needed more than food; she needed attention, safety, security and validation. As she grew in age, she grew in size and emptiness. She said she also grew in anger, resentment, bitterness, misunderstanding, confusion and selfishness. She said if it was negative, she grew in it.

At age 13 and weighing in at more than 200 pounds, she was sent to a secular counselor. She was angry at having to be there. She would often sit through sessions without saying a word. She would hide the car keys or lock herself in a room so she wouldn't have to go, and she got heavier. She stopped getting on the scales at 214 pounds at age 13 because she couldn't handle the reality of who she was and got even heavier.

She said she binged when she could get away with it, when she knew she wouldn't get caught. She would steal candy bars from businesses and food from other people's homes. She was a mess, as bad as any alcoholic or drug user. She was always looking for a good fix.

Sure she purged and sure she hated herself. She said, like every addict, she thought she could stop anytime and go "cold turkey" tomorrow. "That is such a powerful and deceptive lie of the enemy," Brenda says.

Brenda firmly believes every sin is the result of believing a lie, and you can see the lies she believed. She believed the lie that no one had the right to tell her what to do.

She said, on a rare evening with her father when they went out in a boat trolling for fish, her father said something to her she has never forgotten. Her father is not a man of many words. A phone conversation with her father today goes something like this, he will ask, "Are you okay?" She'll say something like, "Yes dad, we are. It's good to hear from you. How are things for you?" "Busy, talk to you soon," and that's it, no hellos, goodbyes, that's it. But this man of few words said something one evening that changed her life. He

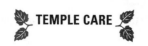

said, "Brennie, you have a choice. You can either keep making yourself and everyone else miserable or you can choose not to. The choice is yours." She wondered if he had been around more would she have gleaned some other nuggets that could have been helpful in her life. She knew she didn't want to be miserable. She had enough misery. So, she chose to do some things that were more socially acceptable, but she still hadn't dealt with the real issue of her unmet needs. She still didn't know Jesus was the answer. She hadn't been introduced to Him yet.

Brenda shared more of her story. It was in college, where she met a woman who seemed so easygoing and at peace with herself that Brenda asked the question every Christian longs to hear: "You're different than others, why?"

The woman brought Brenda to her Bible study, then some church services and soon Brenda knelt down and asked Jesus Christ to be Lord of her life. As her relationship with Jesus grew, her anger, bitterness and resentment lessened and so did her weight. Sure, she restricted her food intake, but this time, she had a Savior who provided a way out from temptation, a Savior who told her not to worry about what to eat or drink, and a Savior who Himself fasted for 40 days. She now had a Savior who provided her victory and it was her choice, as it is yours or anybody else's, whether or not we enter into that victory.

After that session, many of the attendees spoke concerning how much she encouraged and motivated them. Brenda said she believed Biblical counseling can play a significant role in *Temple Care* because it's the truth counteracting the enemy's, the world's and our flesh's deceptive lies. Brenda learned from Neil Anderson that, "you only out truth the enemy, you don't out pray him, wrestle him or trick him."[4] To out truth him and be set free from the strongholds formed against an overeater, you need the truth to make you free. The truth is Jesus.

Both of these testimonies were reprinted with their permission and blessings.

GUIDE TO DUPLICATE THE WORKSHOP

The objective of this project was to address the impending epidemic of obesity in America beginning at home in the local Christian Church. The theory and model presented was *The Relationship of Temple Care to Improved Health for Individuals Afflicted with Obesity*. Biblical knowledge of Temple Care is also the greatest tool for prevention.

As I prayed about the team, I knew it was imperative they had a heart for the obese and a passion to help. God directed me to whom He desired to fill those slots. God handpicked a team of renowned Christian professionals. The team consisted of: Dr. Lisa Hendricks, gynecologist, Dr. Danny Sardon, general surgeon, Dr. Carey Ransone, urologist, Mrs. Brenda Harvey, Biblical Counselor and Dr. Karen Edwards, Naturopath/Herbologist.

This is an excellent project for the congregational nurse, who is presently working in the hospital. I say that because, if your team is not in your congregation, they will be in a health care setting.

I did not receive funding to employ the doctors. Their services were rendered free of charge as a community service, and they are all committed to assist with future workshops because of the need.

The Temple Care Workshop was designated for three weeks (21 days), as previously stated. Again, most research agrees that is the time it takes to create/break and form new lifestyle practices. We met three consecutive Saturdays. The workshops were three hours each Saturday. Time was allotted after each session within that time for questions to be addressed. Each meeting was opened and closed with a prayer. The workshops were recorded.

Food was not served. However, low-fat potluck meals were discussed and encouraged as a part of the workshop. The high-fat meals that are presently being served in the churches are part of the contribution to congregational obesity. We eat and fellowship as often as we can. While continuing to encourage community potluck meals, it is imperative that more tough love is shown by cutting the fat, God said, don't eat it.

The workshop is designed to assist the attendee with understanding what God's Word says about our diet backed with scientific underpinning for better understanding.

One must tailor the workshop to fit the needs of your congregation. In the preparational stages, one should survey the physical disease state of the congregation. Compose a survey which "does not" require a name. List various diseases

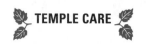

and have time to simply check if they or a family member have it. There would certainly be on your list: high blood pressure, diabetes, cancer and other as it relates to mainly diet. Stress and lack of rest play a major role in the disease process and therefore, must be addressed.

Other organizations assistance will be major. Overeaters Anonymous has a pre-test for one to privately determine if they are addicted to food. If you desire, you can compose a pre and post test. The pre-test determines your churches understanding of what God says about diet before the workshop. The post test will gauge what they have gained as a result of the workshop.

The American Cancer Society gave pocket size books titled *Eat Smart with Fruits and Vegetables* along with many others. The Diabetes Association gave several informative books on diet and diabetes. St. Anthony Memorial gave bags, pens and several give away gift items. I purchased journals and pocket folders along with books that were given away as gift items with the certificate of completion.

I am also a member of the Cancer Care Team at St. Anthony Memorial in Michigan City, IN. Roxy Karnes, the director, came to the workshop and set up a cancer display table which was as professional as a medical convention. There were two palpable models of soft material that was life-like. One model was of a prostate gland with five stages; from normal to stage four inoperable cancer. The purpose was for the men to see and touch what the doctor felt upon digital rectal exam. There was also a model of a breast, so one could palpate to have some idea what a lump would feel like upon breast self exam.

The third model was of the colon, from normal, to a small benign polyp that could easily be snipped during a colonoscopy exam, to stage four cancer. According to most research, obesity contributes to all of the above.

To avoid embarrassment, I placed in each folder a 5X7 ruled index card for private questions they wished to be addressed during the seminar. I had separate pre-registration forms for men and women. The men were having free PSA (Prostate-Specific Antigen) blood testing sponsored by St. Anthony Memorial in Michigan City, IN. Therefore, I needed a head count. The phlebotomists were there to draw blood two hours before the seminar. Actually most of the men were registered by their wives who have an investment in wanting them well. Therefore, the workshop was composed of mainly couples. I encouraged a family support system, especially for teens who usually suffer the pain of obesity, silently.

Male and female pocket folders were stuffed in advance. For example, in the men's folders were *Understanding Prostate Changes* along with other male resources. The ladies packets contained information about breast cancer and diseases related to obesity. Other resources were there for them to select from.

I composed a contract for them to plug in a target weight loss during the workshop. There were weekly weigh-ins, which were actually fun. I encouraged everyone to start with a five pound goal, something achievable. Once the first five is gone it gets easier.

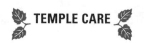

I encourage water aerobics, three times a week, if possible. There are morning and evening classes at your local YMCA or Health Club. The evening class we attended was two days a week, for one hour each. A water aerobics session leaves you feeling as though you've just been massaged.

From the questions that were posed on the 5X7 index cards, I realized for everyone to be comfortable and uninhibited, private sessions were needed with the doctors, for it to be successful. The advertisement for the workshop also addressed the private sessions. The balance of the workshop was coed.

Your marketing will depend on the area you desire to reach. Someone in the congregation advertised the seminar in the faith section of our local newspaper. The church bulletin and sister churches are a good way to advertise at least a month in advance.

Meet with your team to determine what pre-preparation is required for them, before you set your date. Your nutritionist may want them to do a colon cleanse prior to the workshop.

As the coordinator, I was the first presenter. The syllabus was explained and a pre-test was given. They came to each session with excitement, expecting and looking forward to the next one. The first speaker will set the atmosphere for the balance of the workshop.

The private sessions were especially fruitful. Dr. Carey Ransone, urologist and a man of God, was with the men. The men had all of there questions answered that they were ever afraid to ask before. They left the session bouncing as though they were leaving a football game and their team won.

I sat in on the ladies session. All questions were addressed including obesity and pregnancy. Dr. Lisa Hendricks, gynecologist, is also a woman of God. She also addressed the human papilloma virus and the vaccine. She spoke to the many diseases that obesity puts one at risk to. Because of the privacy of the sessions I won't go into detail.

Dr. Danny Sardon, general surgeon, also Christian, spoke to surgical alternatives for those who have not been successful in losing weight by conventional methods, and whose health is dependant on weight loss. He used a power point presentation that showed various types of surgeries. Namely: Gastric bypass, bilio pancreatic diversion and laparoscopic gastric banding. The slide presentation of these different surgeries had illustrations of how they are done and the advantages and disadvantages of the procedures. Counseling pre-surgically and dietary compliance is necessary before and after any of the above named procedures. He went on to explain some of the consequences of obesity which are: reduced life expectancy, increased diseases, physical limitation, social isolation, economic considerations, type II diabetes, hypertension, abnormal fats or lipids in the blood, reflux esophagitis, sleep disorders, asthma, and depression to name a few.

Dr. Karen Edwards, naturopathy/herbologist, is a member of the International Iridology Practitioners Association, American Association of Drugless Practitioners and more. She is the owner of Holistic Alternatives, in LaPorte, IN. "Going back to nature," is her philosophy. She is also a woman of God.

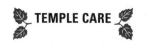

She spoke concerning the importances of undergoing a colon cleanse before starting a new dietary regime. She stressed the individuality of each person's regimen because of different medical issues and medications they may be on and how she worked with medical doctors. Her passion and education is the result of her personal testimony.

Brenda Harvey, Biblical Counselor, member, Association of Christian Counselors, offered Biblical counseling through the workshop. Support groups are needed in the churches, not only for those addicted to drugs and alcohol; they are also needed for food addicts.

Brenda's passion and education were also the outcome of a painful past, as was covered in her testimony. She was 214 lbs at age 13. We are blessed to have her in our church.

Develop a system of reward for those who reach their target weight. I also gave certificates. The gifts I gave were in the form of books. The books were: (1) *Prescription for Nutritional Healing* by Balch, (2) *Alkalize or Die* by Theodore Baroody, (3) a massage book was given to a couple that teaches how to massage each other to relieve stress, and (4) *The New Soul Food* by Fabiala Demps Gains and Roniece Weaver. That book is sponsored by the American Diabetes Association.

Finally, you will find enclosed a printed copy of the power point presentation of my segment of the workshop. The major points are there for you to plug in what's needed to tailor it to your congregation. Remember; be as down to earth as possible. Make it a casual, informal day. May your congregation be blessed as a result of this endeavor.

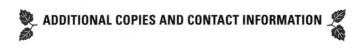

To purchase additional copies please go to:
www.templecaregodsway.com

You may personally contact Rev. Dr. Stephanie Jordan at
www.templecaregodsway.com or
templecareiswisdom@yahoo.com

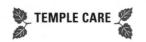# POWER POINT PRINTED VERSION

- <u>Temple</u> — Jesus answered and said to them, Destroy this temple, and in three days I will raise it up. Then the Jews said, "It has taken forty-six years to build this temple , and you will raise it up in three days?" But he was speaking of the temple of his body. (John 2:19-21).

- <u>Care</u> — A big part of the pastoral process. It usually requires an individual plan and usually some type of preparation in advance.

CHURCH

- Church is home away from home for the Christian family to grow in relationship with God and to commune and support each other.

- "There in solitude we recognize our deepest connection with other human beings. The sense of ourselves as religious is enhanced when this social dimension is honored in the Christian setting." —Michael F. Trainer

- Each church body is considered a culture and have their own rituals like different cultures do.

- Some rituals that congregations have are:

  — A particular order of service. Some allow the Holy Spirit to have his way.

  — Pot luck dinners-the food is very tasty and fattening. Healthy, low fat meal should be encouraged.

  — Fellowship Meals

- Although the pot-luck dinners are a great way to come together, too much attention is placed on the meals. These meals may lead to having an obese congregation.

STRESS

- Stress plays a significant role in most addictions.

- The Creator did not design the body to hold stress, and/or toil which came with the fall of humanity (Genesis 3).

- Theodore Baroody defines stress down to the cellular level. He states for best health the body should maintain an "eighty percent alkaline reserve and twenty percent from the acid-forming list."

- Laughter is said to create an alkaline physiological state, which could help alleviate stress.

COUNSELING

- Counseling is an important segment of the healing package.

- A listening presence is imperative in the counseling process.

- Emma Justes, in Hearing Beyond the Words, defines several types or styles of listening.

- One type of listening is Christian Hospitality. It is done with quietness and humility.

SLEEP

- Resting the body is important.

- "Sleep is a sense, and as such is as important to life as seeing, tasting, smelling and hearing. During the sleep period, many acid by-products brought about by over exhaustion, are processed and eliminated from the body through deep breathing and sweating. This repair period is alkaline producing in nature." –Theodore Baroody

- Sleep loss can contribute to obesity.

- The more weight that one gains creates further sleeping problems.

EXERCISE

- According to Neal Barnard, "Exercise is like a giant reset button on your body. It can block your appetite, resets your mood, and puts you in a different relationship with your body."

- Pastors are being encouraged to set up work-out rooms in the churches.

- Exercise increases circulation and helps regulate the immune system and hormones that influence the healing process.

- Those that are obese or morbidly obese have a harder time exercising. Therefore, I recommend water aerobics.

DIET

- According to Dr. Terry Mason, "a diet rich in fruits and vegetables as part of an active lifestyle lowers risk of every diet related disease."

- Kevin Trudeau, author of Natural Cures, is encouraging the public to revert back to natural foods. He states that it is not only overeating, but some of the additives that contributes to obesity.

- "God said, See I have given you every plant-yielding seed that is upon the face of the earth, and every tree with seed in its fruit, you shall have them for food." Gen 1:29

- "The fear and dread of you shall rest on every animal of the earth, and on every bird of the air, on everything that creeps on the ground and on all the fish of the sea; into your hand they are delivered. Every moving thing that lives shall be for food for you; and just as I gave you the green plants, I give you everything. Only you shall not eat flesh with its life, that is, its blood." Gen 9:2-4

- "The Lord spoke to Moses and Aaron, saying to them: Speak to the people of Israel, saying: From the land animals, these are the creatures that you may eat. Any animal that has divided hoofs is cleft footed and chews a cud-such as you may eat. But among those that chew the cud or have divided hoofs, you shall not eat the following: the camel, for even though it chews the cud, it does not have divided hoofs; it is unclean for you. The rock badger, for even though it chews the cud, it does not have divided hoofs; it is unclean for you. The hare, even though it chews the cud, it does not have divided hoofs, it is unclean for you. The pig, for even though it has divided hoofs; and is cleft-footed, it does not chew the cud, it is unclean for you. Of their flesh you shall not eat, and their carcasses you shall not touch; they are unclean for you." Lev 11:1-8

- "Or do you not know that your body is a temple of the Holy Spirit within you, which you have from God, and you are not your own? For you were bought with a price; therefore glorify God in your body." 1 Cor 6:19-20

THE AUTHOR'S TESTIMONY

So shall my Word be that goeth forth out
of my mouth: it shall not return unto me
void, it shall accomplish that which I
please, and it shall prosper in the thing
whereto I sent it.
King James Isaiah 55:11

So will My words that come out of my
mouth not come back empty handed.
They'll do the work I sent them to do,
they'll complete the assignment I gave
them.
Message Bible Isaiah 55:11

The name of Jesus which is the Word, opens the door to the supernatural. Thank God, he honors His Word.

In obedience to "seeking chaplaincy", I enrolled in a clinical pastoral education residency at Christ Hospital and Medical Center in Oak Lawn, Illinois, in September 1993. The morning of the shooting November 8,1993, I was in my office, quietly at my desk preparing for patient rounds.

I heard the voice of God tell me to cancel my 6p.m. dental appointment. Instead of simply picking up the phone and obeying God, I tried to figure out why. To reschedule would have entailed months.

I thought it was my fourteen year old car that two of my three daughters had separate accidents in. As I prayed, I reminded God that he held the car up through my attending Rhema Bible Training Center and back home. Therefore, I was asking Him to keep the car running so it could get me to the dentist. The Holy Spirit kept the car going, it was definitely anointed. I was baptized while driving one day in the Holy Spirit, and prayed in tongues a good percentage of the time I am driving.

So, thinking it was the car, I mapped out a well-traveled street that was a bus-route rather than taking the expressway home. That particular street was only a little over a block walk to my home, in case I had to walk.

The way that I chose, took me through what was considered Chicago's highest crime area, to get to my neighborhood. Somehow, I was not concerned. At that time, I was the assistant pastor to to an inner city church named Faith Bible Center Church, where the Rev. Matthew Perkins was the pastor. The area was well known for gang violence and murder. Our mission was to bring hope, the good news and salvation through Jesus Christ to the broken people and children.

I arrived at peace to my appointment assured that my car was covered with prayer. When I sat in the dentist chair and took a deep breath, I was strongly impressed to read Psalm 91(I read the KJV. The following is the Amplified). I reached into my purse, pulled out my Bible and read it while my dentist was preparing her instruments, then I leaned back into the chair and literally fell sound asleep.

1 He who dwells in the secret place of the Most High shall remain stable and fixed under the shadow of the almighty who's foe no one can withstand.

2 I will say of the Lord, He is my Refuge and my Fortress, my God: on Him I lean and rely, and in Him I confidently trust!

3 For then He will deliver you from the snare of the fowler and from the deadly pestilence.

4 Then He will cover you with His pinions, and under His wings you shall trust and find refuge; His truth and His faithfulness are a shield and buckler.

5 You shall not be afraid of the terror of the night, nor of the arrow, the evil plots and slanders of the wicked that flies by day,

6 Nor of the pestilence that stalks in darkness, nor of the destruction and sudden death that surprise and lay waste at noonday.

7 A thousand may fall at your side, and ten thousand at your right hand, but it shall not come near you.

8 Only a spectator shall you be, yourself inaccessible in the secret place of the Most High as you witness the reward of the wicked.

9 Because you have made the Lord your refuge and the Most High your dwelling place,

10 There shall no evil befall you, nor any plague or calamity come near your tent.

11 For He will give His angels especial charge over you to accompany and defend and preserve you in all your ways of obedience and service.

12 They shall bear you up on their hands, lest you dash your foot against a stone.

13 You shall tread upon the lion and adder; the young lion and the serpent shall you trample underfoot.

14 Because he has set his love upon me, therefore, I will deliver him; I will set him on high, because he knows and understands My name, has personal knowledge of my mercy, love, and kindness-trust and relies on Me, knowing I will never forsake him, no never.

15 He shall call upon Me, and I will answer him; I will be with him in trouble, I will deliver him and honor him.

16 With long life will I satisfy him and show him my salvation

I left the office at 8:30p.m. heading home with that peace that surpasses understanding. As I drove my mind was not on the possibility of danger. I was listening to a Christian talk show while praying in tongues. I wanted to hear soft praise music on the car stereo. I was turning the radio knob while watching the on coming traffic.

Suddenly the terror by night began to unfold in front of my eyes in slow motion as if a TV or drive-in movie screen dropped down in front of me and I was watching it. The on-coming car was heading north bound on the two-lane thoroughfare that was divided by the double yellow line. So, we were an arms length away from each other.

A man was hanging out of the back window, holding what appeared to be a machine gun and wearing a ski mask. He was posed, pointing the gun toward the sky as though he were in a parade.

I simply said, 'Dear Jesus!' and immediately, I clearly felt the impression of an unseen hand on my left shoulder, gently pushing me across my bucket seats toward the passenger side, I know it was the hand of the Lord.

With my left hand still on the steering wheel and my right foot remaining on the gas pedal, I yielded to that gentle push. I didn't consciously think about yielding; I was not in control, I just melted on to the seat like a bowl of warm Jello! God was in control!

As the car was passing, in a split second as I felt the hand of the Lord pushing me down, I heard three gunshots in rapid succession as the gunman fired into my car at close range, aiming at my head. The drivers window of my car was completely shattered. I immediately felt a burning on the left side of my face, and thought that I had been shot. The only word on my lips was the name of Jesus, Jesus, Jesus! I said. "Lord, I hope this is a dream." Nonetheless, I kept repeating the name of Jesus.

Still driving the car, I stayed in that prone position until I was released, no longer feeling the hand. Then feeling dazed, I sat up and looked around to see where I was.

I found later that I had traveled up to a block and a half in that reclined position! The unseen hand guided my car and kept me safely in the flow of traffic, while at the same time, keeping me flat across the bucket seats toward the passenger side.

When I was released to sit up, I was still in the south bound lane, with cars in front and back of me. Everything seemed normal. No one seemed to be aware that anything out of the ordinary had just taken place except the lady behind me.

I honked my horn so that the driver in the car next to me would allow me to turn left into a gas station that was on the corner. The woman in the car behind me also turned into the station, she had seen the entire incident and used her cell phone to call the police. However, as soon as she made sure I had someone to help me, she departed.

The gas station attendants gave me some wet towels to help stop the bleeding on my face. I told them I didn't know if I'd been shot. The burning on the left side of my face made me think a bullet had grazed me. But I just kept saying, 'Jesus! Jesus! Jesus!' I never stopped speaking His name.

Minutes later the police and the ambulance arrived on the scene. While I was being examined by the ambulance driver, I began to feel very hot, so to cool down, I took off the winter tam I was wearing, not realizing at that time that hair came off with it. My hat caught the ambulance drivers attention. He picked it up and asked, "Did you have holes in your hat?" I put my hand on my hip, and answered, "NO", I then stared as he put his fingers through two holes in the hat. There was an entry hole the size of a dime or nickel and an exit hole with a flap the size of a silver dollar. The bullet burned a curl in my hair while penetrating the hat. Meanwhile, the police officer came over and reported that he had examined the car and found a .45 automatic bullet lodged in the front metal window seal on the passenger side.

When I saw his fingers protruding through the holes in the hat, I realized how close I came to getting my head shattered, or blown off. I just began praising the Lord for His deliverance. The ambulance driver and police officer stared at me as if I were a ghost. The police officer exclaimed, "Ma'am, you are lucky!" "No Sir!" I said, "I'm blessed! I'm God's child." I kept shouting praises all the way to the hospital. I came through the emergency room door giving God the glory for what He had done, loudly and shamelessly.

When the medical personnel questioned the nurse about the noise I was making, the nurse answered, "Just leave her alone. That lady has something to shout about!" A short time later, I was released from the hospital after the doctor removed several pieces of glass from the left side of my face. I have the curl that was burned by the bullet and the tam with the holes for a testimony.

When I calmed down, I was reminded that I was disobedient and therefore, repented. I clearly missed God. Praise God, for He had mercy on me. I was talking and praying and not listening to God. So, when I became still, He directed me to His Word and He honored it. His angels are standing at attention waiting for orders from the Word, to perform it!

> Bless the Lord, you His angels,
> who excel in strength, who do
> His Word, Heeding the Voice
> of His Word.
>
> King James Psalms 103:20

The police officer explained that four gang murders had recently taken place near by prior to the attempt on my life. He went on to explain the connection between the two events. He said, "In Chicago, it is becoming increasingly common after a gang murder for gang members to go out looking for an innocent victim to murder as a trophy to celebrate. The police believe that's what was intended in my case. He never left my side as he witnessed God's goodness, and further instructed me that if I must travel that way, don't go through, go around. Even if it's ten miles out of the way to be safe, go around.

I had to fight the spirit of fear for about a month after. Pastor Matthew and his wife Barbara drove me back and forth for a while, as did brother Gregory. A truck backfired one day as my brother was driving, and I hit the floor. We connected at that time because he is a Viet Nam vet who never talked, and he opened up a little with me as a result, simply because I could somewhat relate to being shell shocked. I continued to serve at Faith Bible Center church in the area until 1995, before moving on.

I have shared my testimony as a guest on TV 38's Among Friends, The 700 Club, Sid Roth's Messianic Vision, which is a nationally syndicated Messianic Jewish radio talk show, Christian TV Network in Southfield Michigan, TV 99 in Michigan City, Indiana, Womans Aglow, many churches and Kenneth Hagin Ministries International Word of Faith Magazine. Through the above, millions have been reached with gospel of Jesus.

A SINNER'S PRAYER
To Receive Jesus As Savior

I have heard thy Word through testimony and now realize that without you I can do nothing. I ask forgiveness of my sins and shortcomings and desire thy guiding presence in my life. I thank you for the way you touch the hearts of the willing in a manner that only you can do. I now therefore accept Jesus Christ as my Lord and Savior in accordance with your Word stated in Romans 10:9-10 Amplified.

9 Because if you acknowledge and confess with your lips that Jesus is Lord and in your heart believe (adhere to, trust in, and rely on the truth) that God raised Him from the dead, you will be saved.

10 For with the heart a person believes (adheres to, trusts in, and relies on Christ) and so is justified (declared righteous, acceptable to God) and with the mouth he confesses (declares and openly speaks out freely his faith) and confirms his salvation.

I therefore confess and believe that thou art both Lord and Savior of my life. I am now a member of the family of God. Thank you Lord for saving me!

NOTES

1. Ministry Focus

1. Lewis V. Baldwin, *The Legacy of Martin Luther King Jr.*, (Notre Dame: University of Notre Dame, 2002), 157.

2. *American Obesity Association, Factsheets*, http://www.obesity.org/subs/fastfact/obesity_us.html, 10-04-07, 5:10 p.m.

3. *Major Religions Ranked by Size*, http://www.adherents.com/religions_by_adherents.html, 10-05-07, 5:50 p.m.

4. Sharon Sneed, *The Love Hunger Action Plan*, (Nashville: Thomas Nelson Publications, 1982), 1-2.

5. Major Religions, 1.

6. Ibid.

7. Robert Mathias, *NIDA, Pathological Obesity and Drug Addiction Share Common Characteristics*, volume 16, (October 2001), http://www.drugabuse.gov/NIDA_notes/nnvol16n4/pathological.html, 1.

8. Woman's Health, Milwaukee Journal Sentinel, Nov. 22, 2004, 8:40 p.m., http://www.azcentral.com/health/women/articles/1122obesity-dementia-on.html, 09-01-05.

9. Fern Kazlow, *Making Changes in (No) Time*, http://www.integrateaction.com/article6-html,, 1. 03-07, 1:10 p.m.

10. Pritchett Price, *A Survival Guide to the Stress of Organizational Change* (Dallas: Pritchett and Assoc., 1995), stress.

11. James H. Cone, God of the Oppressed, (Maryknoll:Orbis Books, 2003), 40.

12. Theology of The Missionary Church Government, www.mcncd.org.

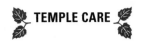

2. Ministry Model

1. Michael F. Trainer, *The Quest For Home, The Household in Mark's Community* (Collegeville: The Liturgical Press, 2001), 3.

2. Tyrone Inbody, *The Faith of the Christian Church* (Grand Rapids: Wm. B. Eerdmans, 2005), 252.

3. Nancy T. Ammerman, Jackson W. Carrol, Carl S. Dudley, and William McKinney *Studying Congregations: A New Handbook* (Nashville: Abingdon Press, 1998), 84.

4. Walter Brueggemann, *The Bible Makes Sense* (Louisville: Westminster John Knox, 2003), 15.

5. Samuel D. Proctor and Gardner C. Taylor, *We Have This Ministry, The Heart of the Pastor's Vocation* (Valley Forge: Judson, 1996), 73-4.

6. Emma J. Justes, *Hearing Beyond the Words* (Nashville: Abingdon, 2006), 10.

7. Peggy Way, *Created By God* (St. Louis: Chalice Press, 2005), 9.

8. Jeff Jay and Debra Jay, *Love First* (Center City: Hazelden, 2000), 3.

9. Ibid., 3.

10. Ibid., 208.

11. Ibid., 95.

12. Ibid., 203.

13. Theodore A. Baroody, *Alkalize or Die* (Waynesville: Holographic Health Press, 2006), 119.

14. William E. Vine, Merrill Unger and William White. *Vine's Expository Dictionary of Old and New Testament Words* (Nashville: Thomas Nelson, 1984).

15. *Encarta World English Dictionary* (New York: St. Martin Press, 1999).

16. Baroody, *Alkalize or Die,* 23.

17. Ibid., 17.

18. Stress-Immune System Health Information, http://www.lifestylelinks.com/stress.htm, 04/14/06, 1.

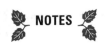

19. Baroody, *Alkalize or Die,* 105.
20. National Public Radio; http://www.NPR.org/templates/story. php?storyid=4206263, (10/30/07).
21. Neal Barnard, *Breaking the Food Seduction* (New York: St Martins Press, 2003), 122.
22. John M. Grohal, "Lack of Sleep Doubles Risk of Obesity," Psych Central   News, http://www.psychcentral.com/news/2006/7/12/lack-or-sleep-doubles-obesity-risk, (10/30/07), 1.
23. Ibid., 1.
24. *Encarta Dictionary.*
25. Krista L. Haines, "Objective Evidence that Bariatric Surgery improves obesity-related obstructive sleep apnea," http://www.galenicom.com/en/medline/article/17349847/all: Murr+MM, (10/30/07), 1.
26. "Regular Exercise Boosts Healing," http://www.archive. newsmax.com/archives/articles/2006/ 4/28/165041.shtml?s= he, (10/31/07 at 5:55a.m.), 1.
27. Ibid., 1.
28. Martha White, *Water Exercise* (Houston: Human Kinetics, 1995), VII.
29. Ibid., 5.
30. "Diabetic-Lifestyle," http://www.diabetic-lifestyle.com/articles/june02_burni_1.htm, (10/31/07 at 5:45a.m.), 3.
31. NCPAD, http://www.ncpad.org/exercise/fat_sheet.php?sheet= 29, (12/01/07 at 9:45p.m.).
32. Terry Mason, "The Role of The Church in Health," assistant Professor of Urology U of I, Commissioner of Health, City of Chicago, Intensive Week Speaker for The United Theological Seminary, January 26, 2006, power point 7.
33. Ibid., power point 1.
34. Ibid.

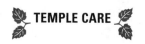

35. Ibid., power point 8.

36. Janet Wagner, "Of Faith and Food," http://www.research.unc.edu/endeavors/ win2001/praise.htm, (11/03/07 at 1:30 p.m.), 1-2.

37. Ibid., collards, 1.

38. Ibid., of Faith and Food, 2.

39. Ibid., collards, 2.

40. Ibid., smaller spoons, 2.

41. Jerome Doolittle, "Bad Attitudes, on Politics, Culture whatever," http://badattitudes.com/ MT/archives/002800.html, (09/01/05 at 3:05 p.m.).

42. Kevin Trudeau, *Natural Cures "They" Don't Want You to Know About* (Elk Grove Village: Alliance, 2004), 86.

43. Ibid.

44. Ibid., 78.

45. Eric Hentges, "National Livestock and Meat Board, and Environmental Nutrition," May 1992, in Sneed, *Love Hunger Action Plan*, 219.

46. Ibid.

47. "Pork Prohibited," http://themusclewoman.com/chooseyour-path/porkprohibited.htm.

48. Louise A. Flood, "Safe From the Flu," http://www.kyrielogy.com/drupal/wwje/safefromtheflu, (10/16/06), 1.

49. Ibid., 2.

50. Louise A. Flood, "To Market To Market to Buy a Fat Hog," http://www.kyrieology.com/ drupal/wwje/tomarket, (10-16-06 at 6:30 p.m.), 3.

51. Ibid.

52. Jean Carper, *The Food Pharmacy* (New York: Bantam Books, 1988), 71.

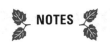

53. Larry Smith, "It's Not Easy Living Clean," *Men's Journal*, vol. XVI no. VL, July 2007, 58.

54. Michael Pollan, "Age of Nutrition," *New York Times Magazine*, January 28, 2007, section 6, 41.

55. Ibid., 44.

3. Biblical Foundation

1. Colin Renfrew, and Katie Boyle, *Archaeogenetics: DNA and the Population Prehistory of Europe* (Oakville: The David Brown Book Co., 2000), 267.

2. Donald K. McKim, *Westminster Dictionary of Theological Terms* (Louisville: Westminster John Knox Press, 1996), "Bible."

3. Ibid.

4. Unless otherwise noted, all scripture references are taken from *The Harper Collins Study Bible, NRSV.* ed., Wayne A. Meeks, (New York: Harper Collins, 1989).

5. Donald L. Migliore, *Faith Seeking Understanding, An Introduction to Christian Theology* (Grand Rapids: Wm. B. Eerdmans, 2004), 47

6. William E. Vine, Merrill Unger and William White, *Vine's Complete Expository Dictionary of Old and New Testament Words* (Nashville: Thomas Nelson, 1985), "soul."

7. McKim, *Westminster Dictionary of Theological Terms*, "spirit," 266.

8. Ibid., "soul, 265," "body, 32."

9. Vine, Unger and White, *Vine's Bible Dictionary*, "Care," 89.

10. Peggy Way, *Created by God* (St. Louis: Chalice Press, 2005), 3.

11. Ibid., 9.

12. Randall Price, *The Temple and Bible Prophecy, A Definitive Look at Its Past, Present and Future* (Eugene: Harvest House, 2005), 138.

13. Ibid., 138.

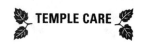
14. *Time Magazine*, October 16, 1989, 64.
15. Vine, Unger and White, *Vine's Bible Dictionary*, "herb."
16. Baroody, *Alkalize or Die*, 23.
17. Custard Apple Nutritional Chart, http://www.custardapple. com/allchart.php
18. Vine, Unger and White, *Vine's Bible Dictionary*, 302.
19. Ibid.
20. Joseph Blenkinsopp, *The Pentateuch, An Introduction to the First Five Books of the Bible* (New York: Doubleday, 1992), 85.
21. Joseph L. Gardner, *Who's Who in the Bible* (China: Readers Digest, 2003), 326 "Noah."
22. John H. Walton, *The NIV Genesis Application Commentary* (Grand Rapids: Zondervan, 2001), 358.
23. R. K. Harrison, *Leviticus an Introduction and Commentary* (Downers Grove: Intervarsity, 1980), 15.
24. Ibid., 16.
25. Roy Gane, *Leviticus and Numbers, the NIV Application Commentary* (Grand Rapids: Zondervan, 2004), 27.
26. Bible footnote under Leviticus 11:1-8.
27. Vine, Unger and White, *Vine's Bible Dictionary*.
28. *Encarta World English Dictionary* (New York: St. Martin Press, 1999).
29. William B. Eerdman, *The Book of Leviticus, The New International Commentary on the Old Testament* (Grand Rapids: Wm. B. Eerdmans, 1979), 172.
30. Ibid., 167.
31. Ibid.
32. Joseph Laffin/Morse, *Funk and Wagnall's New Encyclopedia* vol. 12 (New York: Funk and Wagnall's, 1992), "swine."
33. Henry David Thoreau, "The Vegetarian Way," http://www.homestead.com/dclwolf/ vegetarian.html, 6.

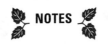

34. Jordan S. Rubin, *The Maker's Diet* (New York: Berkley 2004), 37.

35. Ibid.

36. Gane, *Leviticus and Numbers, The NIV Application Commentary*, 10

37. David Prior, *The Message of 1 Corinthians, The Bible Speaks Today* (Leicesler LEI 7 GP: Inter-Varsity Press, 1992), 103.

38. Emma J. Justes, *Hearing Beyond the Words*.

39. Leon Morris, *Tyndale New Testament Commentaries, 1 Corinthians* (Grand Rapids: Wm B. Eerdmans, 1995), 99-100.

40. Morris, *Tyndale New Testament Commentary, 1 Corinthians*, 95.

41. Tim Dowley, *Eerdmans Handbook to the History of Christianity* (Grand Rapids: William B. Eerdmans, 1988), 198.

42. Ibid.

43. William Webster, "Christian Truths, The Canon; Why Roman Catholic Arguments For The Canon Are Spurious," http://www.freerepublic.com/focus/f.religion/1772346/posts, (10/28/07 at 12:05 p.m.).

44. Ibid., 96.

45. Walter Brueggemann, *An Introduction to the Old Testament, The Canon and Christian Imagination* (Louisville: Westminster John Knox Press, 2003),402

46. Laura Schlessinger and S. Vogel, *The Ten Commandments: The Significance of God's Laws in Everyday Life* (New York: Cleff Street Books, 1998), XXV.

4. Theological Foundation

1. Hosea 4:6

2. McKim, *Westminster Dictionary of Theological Terms*, "human being," 134.

3. 3 John 2

4. Wayne Meeks, *The Harper Collins Study Bible*, foot note under Lev. 11:1-8 (New York: Harper Collins, 1993).

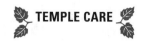

5. R. Cooti, "Review of the Book of Leviticus by Gordon J. Wenham," *Int.* 35 (1981), 423.

6. Ray Gane, *Leviticus/Numbers, The NIV Life Application Commentary* (Grand Rapids: Zondervan, 2004), 23.

7. R. K. Harrison, *Leviticus, An Introduction and Commentary* (Downers Grove: Inter-Varsity Press, 1980), 9.

8. Gane, *Leviticus/Numbers*, 23.

9. Ellen G. White, *The Ministry of Health and Healing* (Nampa: Pacific Press, 2004), 175

10. Ibid., 176.

11. T. Colin Campbell and Thomas M. Campbell II, *The China Study* (Dallas: Ben Bella Books, 2006), 305.

12. R. G. Cassens, *Nitrite-cured meat: a food safety issue in perspective* (Trumbull, CT: Food and Nutrition Press, Inc. 1990).

13. Ibid., 45.

14. Ibid.

15. Ibid., 46

16. Ibid.

17. Ibid.

18. Steven H. Webb, *Good Eating* (Grand Rapids: Brazos Press, 2001), 193

19. Bliss Lentil, "Eat Meat for More, Better Sex," The Peak; http://www.peak.sfu.ca/the-peak/99-3/issue13/meat.html.

20. White, *Ministry of Health and Healing*, 176

21. Daniel Sack, *White-bread Protestants, Food and Religion in American Culture* (New York: Palgrove, 2001), 188.

22. Ibid., 190.

23. Campbell and Campbell, II. *The China Stud*, 52.

24. Dowley, *Eerdmans Handbook of the History of Christianity*, 76-7.

25. Webb, *Good Eating*, 189-90.

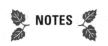

26. "Unani Dietetics: Influence of Food and Drink," Unani Herbal Healing; http://www.unani.com/influence_of_food.htm, (11/18/07 at 12:01).

27. Webb, *Good Eating*, 184-5.

28. Ezekiel 16:49

29. White, *Ministry of Health and Healing*, 99.

30. David Hackett Fischer, *Historian's Fallacies* (New York: Harbor Perennial, 1970), 315.

5. Historical Foundation

1. Reginald Cherry, *The Bible Cure* (Orlando: Creation House, 1998), 1.

2. Ibid., 2-3.

3. McKim, *Westminster Dictionary of Theological Terms*, 129.

4. Jeff Smith, *The Frugal Gourmet Keeps the Feast, Past, Present and Future* (New York: William Morrow and Co., Inc., 1995), 9.

5. Don Colbert, *What Would Jesus Eat* (Nashville: Thomas Nelson, 2002), 18.

6. Smith, *The Frugal Gourmet*, 42.

7. Colbert, *What Would Jesus Eat*, 18.

8. Ibid.

9. Smith, *The Frugal Gourmet*, 9.

10. Marian Maeve O'Brien, *Faith and Food, The Bible Cookbook* (St. Louis: The Bethany Press, 1958), 185.

11. Smith, *The Frugal Gourmet*, 93.

12. *Encarta World English Dictionary*.

13. Cherry, *The Bible Cure*, 76.

14. Smith, *The Frugal Gourmet*, 130.

15. Ronald G. Numbers, *Prophets Of Health: A Study of Ellen G. White* (New York: St. Martin's Press, 2000), 191.

16. Sack, *White Bread Protestants*, 191.

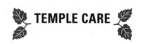
17. Lise Stern, *How to Keep Kosher, a Comprehensive Guide to Understanding Jewish Dietary Laws* (New York: Harper Collins, 2004), 2.

18. Ibid., 5.

19. Ibid., 11.

20. Wayne Daniel Bernard, *When Christians Were Jews* (Cambridge: Cowley Publications, 2006), 105.

21. Cleary, *Qur'an*, 2:168

22. "Egyptian Mummy Shows Taste for Pork," http://www.kriology.com/drupal/www/ egyptmummy, (10/16/06 at 12:15p.m.), 1.

23. Ibid.

24. Bernard, *When Christians Were Jews*, 12.

25. Ibid., 13.

26. Ibid., 113.

27. Walter A. Elwell, *Encyclopedia of the Bible vol. A-1* (Grand Rapids: Baker Book House, 1988), 1143.

28. Naomi Goodman, Robert Marcus and Susan Woolhandler, *The Good Book Cook Book* (New York: Dodd, Mead and Company, 1986), 55.

29. *Eerdman's Dictionary of the Bible* (Grand Rapids: Eerdmans Publishing Co., 2000), food.

30. Smith, *The Frugal Gourmet*, 23.

31. Ibid., 19.

32. "Archeologists re-create The Pompeii Diet," http://www.msnbc.msn.com/id/7980340/, (11/29/07 at 1:50 p.m.), 2.

33. Ibid.

34. Gunther B. Paulien, *The Divine Philosophy and Science of Health and Healing* (Bruhton: Teach Services Inc., 1995), 202.

35. "In Shape Indiana: The Challenge," http://www.in.gov/inshape/challenge/index.html

36. Colbert, *What Would Jesus Eat*, 3.

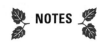

37. Indiana Health Disparities Initiative.

38. Colbert, *What Would Jesus Eat*, 2

39. Lee H. Butler Jr., *A Loving Home* (Cleveland: The Pilgrim Press, 2000), 20.

40. "Soul food," *Wikipedia, the Free Encyclopedia*, http://www.en.wikepedia.org/wiki/soul-food, (04/04/06 at 7:10 a.m.), 1.

41. Ibid.

42. Davis Witt, *Black Hunger* (Minneapolis: University of Minnesota Press, 1999), 80.

43. Cherry, *The Bible Cure*, 20.

44. Anne L. Bower, *African-American Food Ways* (Urbana: University of Ill., 2007), 45.

45. Akbar NA'IM, *Breaking the Chains of Psychological Slavery* (Tallahassee: Mind Productions, 1996), 24.

46. Stern, *How to Keep Kosher*, 109.

47. Ben Lerner, *Body by God* (Nashville: Thomas Nelson, 2003), 5.

48. White, *The Ministry of Health and Healing*, 76.

49. Colbert, *What Would Jesus Eat*.

50. Campbell, *The China Study*, 43.

51. Ibid.

6. Theoretical Foundation

1. Anne H. Soukhanor, *Encarta World English Dictionary*

2. James A. Cone, *God of the Oppressed* (Mary Knoll: Or Books, 2003), 40.

3. Neil T Anderson, Bondage Breaker, Eugene:Harvest House, 1992), crosswalk.com/devotional/dailyinchrist/544556/

4. Ibid.

BIBLIOGRAPHY

Ammerman, Nancy T., Jackson Carroll, Carl S. Dudley, and William McKinney. eds. *Studying Congregations: A New Handbook.* Nashville: Abingdon Press, 1998.

Ault, John. *Nondenominational Church History, Contextual Education.* Michigan City, IN: Countryside Christian Church, 2004.

Baldwin, Lewis V., with Rufus Burrow, Jr., Barbara A. Holmes, and Susan Holmes Winfield. *The Legacy of Martin Luther King, Jr.: The Boundaries of Law, Politics, and Religion.* Notre Dame: University of Notre Dame Press, 2002.

_____. *There Is a Balm in Gilead: The Culture Roots of Martin Luther King, Jr.* Minneapolis: Fortress Press, 1986.

Baroody, Theodore A. *Alkalize or Die.* Waynesville: Holographic Health Press, 2006.

Berard, Wayne-Daniel. *When Christians Were Jews: That is, Now.* Cambridge: Cowley Publications, 2006.

Blenkinsopp, Joseph. *The Pentateuch: An Introduction to the First Five Books of the Bible.* New York: Doubleday, 1992.

Booth, Wayne C., Gregory G. Calomb, and Joseph M. Williams. *The Craft of Research.* Chicago: University of Chicago Press, 1995.

Bower, Anne L. *African American Food warp: Explorations of History and Culture.* Urbana: University of Illinois Press, 2007.

Brueggemann, Walter. *The Bible Makes Sense.* Louisville: Westminister John Knox, 2001.

_____. *An Introduction to the Old Testament: The Canon and Christian Imagination.* Louisville: John Knox, 2003.

Butler, Lee H., Jr. *A Loving Home: Caring For African-American Marriage and Families.* Cleveland: The Pilgrim Press, 2000.

Campbell, T. Colin and Thomas M. Campbell II. *The China Study: Startling Implications for Diet, Weight-loss and Long Term Health.* Dallas: Ben Bella Books, 2006.

Canton, Patricia. *Professional Development as Transformative Learning: New Perspective for Teachers of Adults.* San Francisco: Jossey Bass, 1996.

Carper, Jean. *The Food Pharmacy: Dramatic New Evidence That Food is Your Best Medicine.* New York: Bantam Books, 1989.

Cherry, Reginald. *The Bible Cure.* Orlando: Creation House, 1998.

Cleary, Thomas. *The Qur'an: A New Translation.* Chicago: Starlatch Press, 2004.

Colbert, Don. *What Would Jesus Eat? The Ultimate Program for Eating Well, Feeling Great and Living Longer.* Nashville: Thomas Nelson, 2002.

Cone, James. *God of the Oppressed.* Maryknoll: Orbis Books, 2003.

Creswell, John W. *Research Design: Qualitative, Quantitative and Mixed Method Approaches. 2nd Edition.* Thousand Oaks: Sage, 2003.

Davies, Richard E. *Handbook for Doctor of Ministry Projects: An Approach to Structured Observation of Ministry.* Lanham: University Press of America, 1984.

Doolittle, Jerome. *Bad Attitudes, on Politics Culture, Whatever.* http://www.badattitudes.com/mt/archives/002800.html, 09/01/05, 3:05.

Dowley, Tim. *Eerdmans Handbook of the History of Christianity.* Grand Rapids: William B. Eerdmans, 1988.

Eerdmans, William B. *The Book of Leviticus: The New International Commentary on the Old Testament.* Grand Rapids: William B. Eerdmans, 1979.

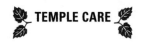 **TEMPLE CARE**

Eerdmans Dictionary of the Bible. Grand Rapids: Eerdmans Publishing Co., 2000.

Elwell, Walter A. *Encyclopedia of the Bible, vol. A-1*. Grand Rapids: Baker Book House, 1988.

Encarta World English Dictionary. New York: St. Martin Press, 1999.

Fischer, David H. *Historian's Fallacies Toward a Logic of Historical Thought*. New York: Harper Perennial, 1970.

Gane, Roy. *Leviticus and Numbers: The NIV Commentary*. Grand Rapids: Zondervan, 2004.

Gardner, Joseph L. *Who's Who in the Bible*. China: Reader's Digest, 2003.

Goodman, Naomi, Robert Marcus and Susan Woolhandle. *The Good Book Cookbook: Recipes From Biblical Times*. New York: Dodd, Mead and Co., 1986.

Greenwood, Davydd J. and Morton Levin. *Introduction to Action Research: Social Research for Social Change*. Thousand Oaks: Sage Publications, 1998.

Harrison, R. K. *Leviticus an In Introduction and Commentary*. Downer Grove: Intervarsity, 1980.

Herald Argus. "Hoosiers Losing the Battle of the Bulge." LaPorte, Indiana Newspaper, front page. May 25, 2006.

Inbody, Tyrone. *The Faith of the Christian Church: An Introduction to Theology*. Grand Rapids: William B. Eerdman, 2005.

Jay, Jeff and Debra Jay. *Love First: A New Approach to Intervention for Alcoholism and Drug Addiction*. Center City: Hazelden, 2000.

Justes, Emma J. *Hearing Beyond the Words: How to Become a Listening Pastor*. Nashville: Abingdon Press.

Laffin, Joseph/Morse, Funk, Wagnalls. *New Encyclopedia, vol. 12*. New York: Funk and Wagnalls, 1992.

Lerner, Ben. *Body by God*. Nashville: Thomas Nelson Publishers, 2003.

Mann, Thomas. *A Guide to Library Research Methods.* New York: Oxford University Press, 1990.

Mason, Terry. *The Role of the Church in Health.* Assistant Professor of Urology, U of I Commissioner of Health, city of Chicago, United Theological Seminary Intensive lunch lecture, Wednesday, January 26, 2006, handout.

McKim, Donald. *Westminister Dictionary for Theological Terms.* Louisville: Westminister John Knox, 1996.

McNibb, Jean, Pamela Lomax and Jack Whitehead. *You and Your Action Research Project.* New York: Routledge Farmer, 2003.

Meeks, Wayne A. *The Harper Collin's Study Bible NRSV.* New York: Harper Collins, 1993.

Meyers, William R. *Research in Ministry: Primer for the Doctor of Ministry Program. 3rd Edition.* Chicago: Exploration Press ©2000,2002.

Migliore, Daniel L. *Faith Seeking Understanding: An Introduction to Christian Theology. 2nd Edition.* Grand Rapids: William B. Eerdman's, 2004.

Miles, Matthew B. and A. Michael Huberman. *Qualitative Data Analysis: An Expanded Source book. 2nd Edition.* Thousand Oaks: Sage Publications, 1994.

Morris, Joseph L. *Funk and Wagnall's New Encyclopedia. vol. 12.* New York: Funk and Wagnall's, 1992.

Morris, Leon. *Tyndale New Testament Commentaries.* Grand Rapids: William B. Eerdman, 1995.

Musser, Donald W. & Joseph L. Price, eds. New & Enlarged Handbook of Christian Theology. Nashville: Abingdon Press, 2003.

NA'IM, Akbar. *Breaking the Chains of Psychological Slavery.* Tallahassee: Mind Productions, 2006.

Numbers, Ronald G. *Prophets of Health: A Study of Ellen White.* New York: St. Martin's Press, 2000.

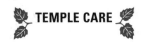 **TEMPLE CARE**

O'Brien, Marian Maeve. *Faith and Food: The Bible Cookbook.* St. Louis: The Bethany Press, 1958.

Paulien, Gunther B. *The Divine Philosophy and Science of Health and Healing.* Bruhton: Teach Services Inc., 1995.

Pohley, Kenneth. *Transforming the Rough Places: The Ministry of Supervision. 2nd Edition.* Franklin: Providence House Publishers, 2001.

Pollan, Michael. *Unhappy Meals.* New Times Magazine, January 28, 2007.

Price, Randall. *The Temple and Bible Prophecy: A Definitive Look at It's Past, Present and Future.* Eugene: Harvest House, 2005.

Prior, David. *The Message on 1 Corinthians, the Bible Speaks Today.* Leicesler LEI 7 GP: Intervarsity Press, 1992.

Pritchett, Price. *A Survival Guide to the Stress of Organizational Change.* Dallas: Pritchett and Assoc., 1995.

Proctor, Samuel. *The Substance of Things Hoped For: A Memoir of African-American Faith.* Valley Forge: Judson Press, ©1995, 1999.

Proctor, Samuel, and Gardner C. Taylor. *We Have This Ministry: The Heart of the Pastors Vocation.* Valley Forge: Judson, 1996.

Renfrew, Colin and Katie Boyle. *Archaeogenetics: DNA and the Population Prehistory of Europe.* Oakville: The David Brown Book Co., 2000.

Rubin, Jordan S. *The Maker's Diet: The 40-day Health Experience That Will Change Your Life Forever.* New York: The Berkeley Publication Group, 2004.

Sack, Daniel. *White Bread Protestants.* New York: Palgrove, 2000.

Schlessinger, Laura and S. Vogel. *The Ten Commandments: The Significance of God's Laws in Everyday Life.* New York: Cleff Street Books, 1998.

Smith, Jeff. *The Frugal Gourmet Keeps the Feast: Past, Present and Future.* New York: William Morrow and Co., Inc., 1995.

Smith, Larry. "It's Not Easy Living Clean." *Men's Journal* vol. XVI no. VL, July 2007.

Sneed, Sharon. *The Love Hunger Action Plan*. Nashville: Thomas Nelson Publications, 1982.

Stern, Lise. *How to Keep Kosher: A Comprehensive Guide to Understanding Jewish Dietary Laws*. New York: William Morrow, 2004.

Tanakh, The Jewish Bible. Philadelphia: The Jewish Publication Society, 1985.

Thomas, Owen C. and Ellen K. Wondra. *Introduction to Theology*. 3rd *Edition*. Harrisburg: Morehouse Publications, 2002.

Tiffany, Fredrick C. and Sharon H. Ringe. *Biblical Interpretation: A Road Map*. Nashville: Abingdon Press, 1996.

Trainer, Michael F. *The Quest for Home, the Household in Marks Community*. Collegeville: The Liturgical Press, 2001.

Trudeau, Kevin. *Natural Cures "They" Don't Want You to Know About*. Elk Grove Village: Alliance Publishing Group, 2004.

Vine, William E., Merrill Unger Frederick and William White. *Vine's Expository Dictionary of Old and New Testament Words*. Nashville: Thomas Nelson, 1984.

Walton, John H. *The NIV Genesis Application Commentary*. Grand Rapids: Zondervan, 2001.

Way, Peggy. *Created by God: Pastoral Care for All God's People*. St. Louis: Chalice Press, 2005.

Webb, Steven H. *Good Eating*. Grand Rapids: Brazo Press, 2001.

White, Ellen G. *The Ministry of Health and Healing: An Adaptation of Ellen White's Classic Work, the Healing In Today's Language*. Nampa: Pacific Press, 2004.

White, Martha. *Water Exercise*. Houston: Human Kinetics, 1995.

Witt, Doris. *Black Hunger*. Minneapolis: University of Minnesota Press, 1999.

Wolcott, Harry F. *Writing Up Qualitative Research*. Newbury Park: Sage Publications, 1990.

ONLINE SOURCES

American Diabetes Association. "Soul Food Gets a Facelift." http://www.lendeversity.com/villages/africa/arts-culture-media-bpr- soulfood0604.asp; 21 September 2006

American Obesity Association Fact Sheet http://www.obesity.org/subs/ fastfact/obesity_us.html. 4 October 2007

Custard Apple Nutritional Chart. http://www.custardapple.com.all/chart.php. 10/16/06, 8:30 a.m.

Diabetic-Lifestyle. http://www.diabetic-lifestyle.com/artcles/june02_burni_1.htm, 10/31/07, 5:45 p.m.

Egyptian Mummy Shows Taste for Pork. http://www.krieology.com/drupal/ www/ egyptmummy, 10/16/16,12:15 p.m.

Flood, Louise A. *To Market, to Market to Buy a Fat Hog.* http://www.kyrielogy.com/drupal/wwje/tomarket, 10/16/06, 6:30 p.m.

Grohal, John M., Psy.D. *Lack of Sleep Doubles Risk of Obesity.* http://www.psychcentral .com/news/2006/7/12/lack-of-sleep-doubles-obesity-risk.html, 10/30/07.

Haines, Krista L. *Objective Evidence that Bariatric Surgery Improves Obesity Related Obstructive Sleep Apnea.* http://www.galeni-com.com /en/medicine/article 17349847/all:murr+mm, 10/30/07.

Health Services Use and Health Costs of Obese and Non-Obese Individuals. http://www.*archinterumed*.com@Indiana School of Medicine, 10/16/05, 8:10am.

In Shape Indiana: The Challenge. http://www.in.gov/inshape/challenge/index.html.

Kazlow, Fern. *Making Changes in (NO) Time.* http://www.itegrativeaction.com/ article6.html.

Major Religions Ranked by Size. http://www.adherents.com/religions_by_adherents.html.

Mathias, Robert. *Pathological Obesity and Drug Addiction Share Common Brain Characteristics, volume 16, number 4* (Oct. 2001). http://www.drugabuse.gov/NIDA-notes/NNVvol16N4/pathological.htm, 10/16/06, 2:15 p.m.

NCPAD. http://www.ncpad.org/exercise/fat_sheet.php?sheet=29, 12/01/04, 9:45 p.m.

Neighmond,   Patricia. http://www.NPR.org/templates/story.php?storyid=4206263, 10/30/07.

Obesity. http://www.weightlossobesity.com/obesity/obesity.html, 2, 04/12/06, 3:15 p.m.

Obesity Statistics Related to Overweight and Obesity. http://www.weightlossobesity.com/ obesity/overwieght-and-obesity-statistics.html, 04/12/06, 3:03 p.m.

Regular Exercise Boosts Healing. http://www.archive.newsmax.com/archives/articles/ 2006/4/28/165041.shtml?=he, 10/31/07, 5:55am.

Soul Food Widepedia, The Free Encyclopedia, http://www//en.widepedia.org/WIFI/soul-food, 08/22/06, 1:18.

Stress Immune System Health Information. http://www.lifestylelinks.com/stress.htm, 04/14/06.

Stress and It's Control on You! http://www.biotanicalchi.com/aboutstress.html, 04/14/06, 1:30 p.m.

Thoreau, Henry David. *The Vegetarian Way.* http://www.homestead.com/dclwolf/ vegetarian.html.

Wagner, Janet. *Of Faith and Food.* http://www.research.unc.edu/endeavors/win2001/ praise.htm, 11/03/07, 1:30 p.m.

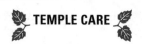

TEMPLE CARE

Webster, William. *Christian Truth, The Canon: Why the Roman Catholic Arguments for the Canon are Spurious.* http://www.freepublic.com/focus/f.religion/1772346/ posts, 09/28/07, 12:05.

Woman's Health, Milwaukee Journal Sentinel. http://www.azcentral.com/health/ womans/articles/1122obesity-dementia-on.html, 09/01/05, 8:40.